AF422118

Know Thy
SOUND

JAY GIBSON

ISBN: 979-8-227-28092-3 (Paperback)
ISBN: 979-8-9908969-1-8 (eBook)

Cover design: Marta Šušić (Obućina)
Editing: Michelle Gean (michelle@bookwritingaccelerator.com)
Illustration: Marta Šušić (Obućina)
Interior design and formatting: Nonon Tech & Design

Available on Amazon and other retail outlets.

TABLE OF CONTENTS

Disclaimer 1

Acknowledgements 3

Chapter 1: A Journey into the World of Sound Healing 5
Overview 5
Comprehension 9
Therapy 13
Homeostasis 17
Cymatics 21
Intention 25

Chapter 2: Exploring the past/Coloring book 33
History 33
Ancient Greece 36
Viking 38
China 39
Egypt 41
India 42
Italy 43
America 44
Africa 46
Australia 47
Mexico 49

Oldest Instrument 51
Modern Times 51
Weaponized Sound 53
Fantasy 54
Recommendations 55

Chapter 3: Singing Bowl Differences 59
Mesopotamia 59
Bon Culture of Tibet 60
Ancient Bowls and Metals 62
The Rise of the Quartz Bowl 66
Crystal Alchemy Bowls™ 69
Super Grades™ 74

Chapter 5: Energy Centers 77
Chakras 77
Brief History 79
Singing bowls 80
Root Chakra 82
Sacral Chakra 86
Solar Plexus Chakra 88
Heart Chakra 90
Throat Chakra 93
Third Eye Chakra 96
Crown Chakra 99
Chakra Frequencies 102
Chakra Cleansing and Purification Exercise 103
Endocrine System 106
The Reproductive Glands C# 108
The Adrenal Glands D# 109
Thyroid Gland G# 111
The Pineal Gland A# 112

High Crown...113

Precautions...114

Chapter 6: Sounds of Theory 117

Introduction 117

Frequencies and Notes...118

Sharps and Flats 122

Scales 123

Keys 128

Triads and Chords..130

Chord Progressions 131

Tuning Standards 135

Building the Ideal Set for You 140

Octaves..141

Ideology 143

Credits 144

Chapter 7: Crating sets 147

What are Sets 147

Why is Building Sets Important 147

Types of Sets...148

Set Building Strategies...162

Guidelines to Follow While Building 163

3 Bowl Sets 165

5 Bowl Sets Following the Pentatonic Scale. 167

Majors 167

Minors 168

Cultural Pentatonic Scales...169

Zodiac Sign Pentatonic Scales 170

Deity Pentatonic Scales...172

Pentatonic Scales for the Seasons...............................174

7 Bowl Sets 175

Singing Bowls with World Melodies 186

Lullabies 189

Brahms' Lullaby (Wiegenlied: Guten Abend, gute Nacht) 190

Hymns 193

Raghupati Raghav Raja Ram 193

Folk Songs 195

Scarborough Fair 196

Bonus 199

Durin's Song 199

How to Play a Crystal Bowl 203

Chapter 8: Safety, Consent, and Post-Session
        Support 215

My First Sound Bath 215

Mount Shasta 218

Energy 220

Direction 222

Clear Intention 225

Barriers 225

Precautions 226

Aftercare 230

About the Author 263

DISCLAIMER

Despite all the miraculous things witnessed with sound healing and Singing bowls. The content within this book is not a substitute for professional medical advice, diagnosis, or treatment.

The information provided here is for educational and for informational purposes only. It should not be used as a replacement for consultation with a qualified healthcare professional.

The use of Singing bowls and related practices should be approached with care and caution, and individuals with pre-existing medical conditions or those who are currently under medical treatment should seek guidance from their healthcare providers before incorporating these practices into their wellness routines.

The author and publisher of this book do not assume responsibility for any consequences arising from the use of the information presented herein.

By reading this book, you acknowledge and agree to the terms of this disclaimer and understand that it is your responsibility to make informed choices regarding your health and wellness.

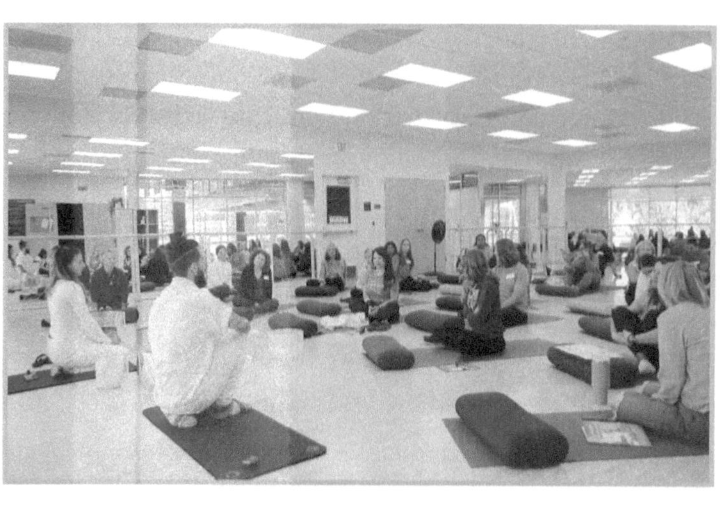

ACKNOWLEDGEMENTS

A deserved thank you to Crystal Tones®, without the opportunity they provided, this book would not exist. From a young age, I was drawn to Eastern philosophy, chakras, metaphysics, and all things esoteric and holistic, exploring different techniques and lifestyle choices to incorporate and teach. However, my journey with Crystal Tones® ignited the flame and compelled me to go deeper and create this body of work. Working with Crystal Tones® was always a test and a blessing. The challenges and hurdles that could arise internally and externally pushed me to grow and evolve. The owners didn't always give me easy answers, transforming me further into a seeker and deepening my knowledge and understanding. This book is not just a personal endeavor but a testament to the countless individuals I continue to interact with daily who seek practical answers that can now be found within these pages. I also want to express my heartfelt gratitude and dedicate this book to all the writers who have paved the way in this subject. Their contributions and insights have been invaluable, shaping the landscape of knowledge and understanding. Throughout this book,

I mention various works I have enjoyed reading that left a lasting impression on me. The diversity of perspectives and the many specific techniques covered in these books have greatly enriched my understanding. I would like to extend my sincere appreciation to my brother Cody. His honesty, genuine support, and unconditional love has always been a constant source of strength and encouragement throughout this endeavor. I am incredibly grateful to the team I managed at Crystal Tones®. Their inquisitive minds, thought-provoking questions, and eagerness to learn fueled my passion and enriched the content of this book. I also want to acknowledge and thank Quorra, who stands as one of the world's finest Singing bowl set builders. Their exceptional talent and dedication provided me with healthy competition, driving to push beyond any self-limiting beliefs. Last but certainly not least, I want to express my deepest gratitude to the caretakers of my son. Your selflessness, dedication, and support have been instrumental in allowing me the availability for this creative journey.

Chapter 1

A JOURNEY INTO THE WORLD OF SOUND HEALING

OVERVIEW

If there's one thing I want everyone to take away from this book, it's this: Using sound to heal has depth and layers but it's not something that is only accessible to the rich, spiritually gifted, secret societies, people with degrees or that deeply study the subject. It's actually a lot more simple and if practiced can easily be understood and applied to the daily lives of everyone. This book is intended to guide your journey into the world of sound; it's to be used as a curriculum for new or seasoned practitioners.

Let me give you a simple example.

Imagine we're conversing, sharing thoughts, I start yelling, banging something or even use a condescending tone. All those sounds produce certain emotions inside of you. In contrast, consider us having a positive dialogue beside a gentle, flowing river. It's the soothing, restorative qualities of certain sounds that hold the key.

Not all sounds possess a "healing potential," just as not all foods contribute to our health. It's the same with all of our senses and being mindful. The things we take in through all of our senses either work to help our systems or they work against them.

The purpose of this book is to help educate and inform about sound and how it can help us find health, and balance in our lives.

Sound as a healing modality dates back thousands of years, and its effectiveness has been documented across various cultures and religions. Sound possesses the ability to transcend the barriers of language and belief systems. It speaks directly to the core of our being, bypassing the limitations of words and cultural differences. Just as our other senses — sight, taste, touch, and smell — shape our perception of the world, the sounds we encounter have an impact.

In contrast, exposure to discordant or harmful sounds can disrupt our equilibrium and lead to various forms of stress and disease. The negative impact of noise pollution on our physical, emotional, and mental well-being is also well-documented.

All you have to do is walk around a city, and you can hear the chaos that we have normalized. Whether you realize it or not, it's taking a toll.

The use of sound for therapeutic purposes is not just a recent trend but has been documented in ancient texts, hieroglyphs, and mythology worldwide. From the mesmerizing chants of early Roman Gregorian monks to the rhythmic vibrations of didgeridoos and drums resonating in the Australian tribes and the enchanting descriptions of the sacred Indian Vedas, they understood that sound has the innate ability to harmonize, entrain, and restore balance within us.

From the Bible to numerous early texts, schools of ancient Egypt, Masons, Rosicrucian's etc have all delved deep into the realm of sound for spiritual and physical healing. These threads of wisdom, woven through time, bear witness to the universality of sound as a tool embraced by diverse cultures across the earth.

Sound, throughout history, has been known not only for its healing properties but also for its capacity to bring destruction.

I personally love quotes, movie one liners and any type of short sentence or statement that captures an idea and provokes one to think.

Here are some early references from the bible and the vedas on regards to the power of sound:

BIBLE

*"Praise him according to his excellent greatness!
Praise him with trumpet sound; praise him with lute
and harp!"* - Psalm 150:1-3

*"And I will cause the noise of your songs to cease,
and the sound of your lyres shall be heard no more."* -
Ezekiel 26:13

*"And the Lord will cause his majestic voice to be
heard and the descending blow of his arm to be seen,
in furious anger and a flame of devouring fire, with a
cloudburst and storm and hailstones."* - Isaiah 30:30

VEDAS

*"He who sings with melody measures the earth and
heaven with his song."* - Atharvaveda 6.13.1

*"Through sound, speech, and hymns, may all beings
be happy."* - Atharvaveda 19.9.5

*"Through the power of sound, the gods create and
sustain the universe."* - Rigveda 10.121.5

As you can see, these selected references represent a glimpse of countless writings highlighting the power and significance of sound.

With technological advancements and the spread of information, people are rediscovering the power of sound as a holistic approach to healing and therapy. Whether you are a fan of ancient myths and legends or a lover of science and innovation, sound healing offers something for everyone.

Comprehension

Personally and professionally, I have had the privilege of witnessing and being a part of hundreds of sound baths, If you don't know what a sound bath is, there is a variety of variations but typically what you see these days is a group of people laying down for a half hour to a hour while you have the host playing different instruments, a single instrument or even just using their voice. The host is using sound to facilitate an environment that will promote healing through relaxation, if you understand the body's nervous system this makes more sense.

Working for Crystal Tones® and Seeing thousands of Crystal Alchemy Singing Bowls find homes worldwide, and working with individuals from all walks of life, including esteemed NASA engineers, doctors, children, animals, the elderly, addicts, energy-sensitive individuals and people who have no experience whatsoever. Witnessing the effects of sound on individuals from diverse backgrounds, regardless of language, profession, or education, has been a truly remarkable experience to be a part of.

> *"Music is a higher revelation than all wisdom and philosophy."* - Ludwig van Beethoven.

To explore sound healing, let's start with a simple way to comprehend and understand what it is: Sound healing is a practice that uses the power of sound waves to support the restoration of our being back to a state of homeostasis. It works on the principle of entrainment, where the vibrations of specific sounds synchronize with our body's natural rhythms. Just as certain sounds can induce a sense of relaxation and calmness, the jarring and intense beats of loud war drums etc can create chaos and unease. By continually and consciously surrounding ourselves with peaceful and harmonious sounds, we create an environment that promotes our health and rejuvenation. The Frequencies can help entrain our cells back to how they function optimally, versus other frequencies that can fragment the perfect geometry within us.

By using various instruments and techniques, such as crystal singing bowls, tuning forks, gongs, and chanting, sound healers aim to stimulate the body's natural healing mechanisms.

This quote is overused, but it's the truth and deserves a spotlight:

> *"To find the universe's secrets, think about energy, frequency, and vibration."*
> — Nikola Tesla

The practitioner uses various techniques to produce specific sounds and vibrations during a sound healing session. The recipient can experience the sounds and vibrations through their ears and by feeling the vibrations in their body. If you've ever attended a loud concert or experienced the booming sound system in certain movie theaters, you've likely felt how the bass can reverberate through your entire body. This is a tangible example of how sound waves and vibrations can affect us. Our bodies literally respond to these vibrations, and understanding the relationship between the sound and our bodies can deepen our awareness of how sound influences our health and experiences.

Most humans have the ability to perceive sounds within the frequency range of approximately 20-30 Hz up to 15-20kHz. What adds a dimension to this auditory spectrum is the fact that certain overtones, undertones, and harmonics produced by Singing bowls can extend beyond or fall below this range. Although these frequencies may go unheard by our ears, our skin, being the body's largest organ, is capable of sensing and absorbing them. Our body will notice the slightest cent change before our ears. This contributes to the experience of being in the presence of Singing bowls, particularly when compared to listening to audio recordings. The limitation in the audio recording equipment, especially if it is of lower quality, as it may selectively capture only a specific range of hertz, often neglecting a significant portion of the nuanced sounds or compressing them to a flat and lifeless rendition. The playback device and the type of earphones used further influence the overall perception of the sounds.

Research has shown that sound healing can help reduce stress and anxiety, promote relaxation, improve sleep, boost immune function, reduce pain and inflammation, improve mood, and enhance cognitive function. There are hundreds of books on the subject now, I will list some of my favorites later on. There is also a good amount of positive case studies posted by the natural library of medicine. I suggest checking out their website if diving into case studies is your thing.

Moreover, sound healing has also been found to be effective in helping to treat a wide range of physical and mental health conditions, such as depression, anxiety, PTSD, chronic pain, and even cancer. It is important to emphasize that consulting with a healthcare professional like your doctor is always a wise and recommended step. While many aspects of life can be approached from a preventative standpoint, it is essential to recognize that prevention does not guarantee a cure. Likewise, while specific approaches may be effective treatments, they cannot ensure absolute success. When dealing with serious matters, seeking medical professional assistance and guidance is always advisable, it also starts with your own personal belief that you can and will heal.

I recall a talk on youtube by Sadguru, where he made a joke on the importance of seeking medical assistance when necessary. He mentioned that holistic and preventative activities like yoga, diets, mantras and taking certain herbs and remedies can promote health. One can even pray and ask for divine intervention. However, he emphasized that even with all these efforts, reciting a mantra won't save you if your leg is broken and your bone is hanging out bleeding everywhere. At that point you need to go to the doctor. The analogy made me laugh, but it's true.

Overall, sound healing offers a non-invasive and holistic approach to healing that has been practiced for thousands of years and is gaining more recognition and acceptance in modern medicine and science.

THERAPY

I want to take a closer look at the concept of therapy in the context of sound healing.

Therapy, also known as treatment or intervention, involves caring for and assisting individuals with medical, mental health, or other conditions. It can address various issues, including physical health problems, mental health conditions, developmental disabilities, and behavioral issues.

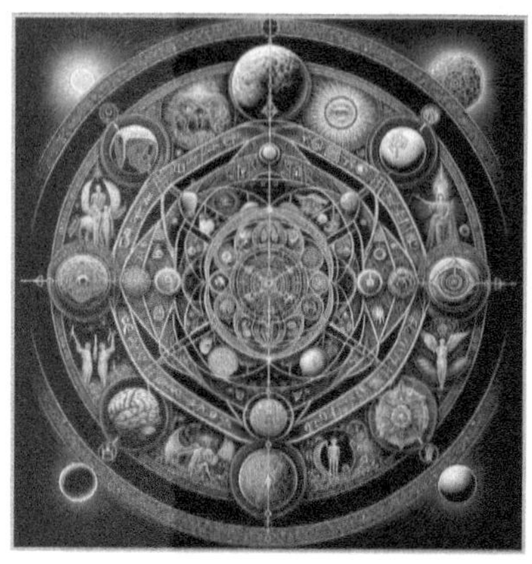

It is also important to remember that the healing process can be challenging and usually is. Despite the glamorization of spirituality in modern times, people may have deep-seated triggers, traumas, or issues that they have consciously or unconsciously repressed for a very long time. Be aware that certain sounds, tastes, or smells may trigger these responses, as we all have memories tied to our senses that vary from person to person.

I personally suffer from vasovagal syncope which I believe is based on a trigger which I feel was created when I was 12 when I had to watch my mom overdose. To this day when I see people that are pale in the hospital or when I see blood I tend to faint. When working on someone to try and heal them you should always be cautious and as informed as you can on what might trigger them. At least provide the safest space possible for them to have that release.

One aspect of Sound healing is that it can help individuals enter the same brain states used in hypnotherapy, which is a type of therapy that utilizes hypnosis, a form of deep relaxation, to access the unconscious mind to reprogram and promote positive changes in thoughts, feelings, behaviors, and the individuals narrative around certain triggers.

The effects of sound healing can vary depending on an individual's journey through life, the type of sounds and vibrations used, the instruments and environment, and whether the person is lying down, sitting, or standing. It is not uncommon for people to fall asleep. On the other hand, they may experience intense emotions during sound healing sessions, such as crying, anger, relief, or even sexual stimulation. As such, it is important to approach sound healing with mindfulness and respect for its potential impact.

When I started practicing sound healing, I didn't fully understand the importance of providing proper before or aftercare. As a result, some of my sessions ended up bringing up a lot of unresolved emotions and triggering memories for myself and my clients without providing them with a healthy way to process these experiences post session. Additionally, conducting sound healing sessions could leave me feeling exhausted, which is something we will delve into more later on.

Sound healing sessions can take on many different forms and serve various purposes. Some people use them for guided meditations or channeling work, while others may work with clients struggling with addiction or other mental health issues and trying to work through releasing those traumas. The possibilities are limitless and only bounded by the imagination and intention of the practitioner.

The power of sound and creation itself is at the heart of sound healing. Even our self-narrative and how we speak to ourselves daily is a prime example of this. Negative self-talk can impact our mental, physical, and emotional health, while positive affirmations can help cultivate feelings of gratitude, hope, and possibility. As such, sound healing is a reminder that the power of healing begins with ourselves and the way we use our voices and intentions to shape our reality.

"The human voice is the most beautiful instrument of all, but it is the most difficult to play."
- Maya Angelou.

When introducing someone to sound healing for the first time, create a comfortable and safe environment. Rather than diving into the intricacies and all the technicalities, it's best to start with a simple demonstration using a Singing bowl or a handheld practitioner bowl. The goal is to get the person to feel and experience sound, rather than overloading them with complex information.

Less in the head, more in the heart

To begin, I often ask the person to close their eyes and take a few deep breaths to release any anxiety or tension they may be holding. I then introduce the Alchemy bowl or practitioner bowl and instruct them to focus on the sound and follow their breath as they deeply but gently inhale and exhale through the nose. I play the bowl gently. Once the bowl starts to sing, I take the mallet off and let it fade out, you don't want to overplay it here as overplaying can cause a dissonance and also lead to bowls breaking. After a few minutes, I thank them and ask them to open their eyes. I have never had anyone tell me they felt nothing during the short session. Even this limited experience can create a sense of peace and calm, slow the heart rate, and help to restore balance. This brief introduction aims to help the person have a personal experience.

HOMEOSTASIS

One of the principles of sound healing is the concept of homeostasis, which refers to the body's ability to maintain a stable, balanced internal environment in response to changes in the external environment. This process is paramount for the proper functioning of the body's systems and organs, and homeostasis disruptions can lead to various health problems. Sound healing can help to restore homeostasis by introducing the proper frequencies and vibrations into the body. Every body part, from our cells to our organs, has a specific frequency that should resonate for optimal health. When we are exposed to things that disrupt or distort these frequencies, such as stress, unhealthy and processed foods, endocrine disruptors, etc., our body's systems can become imbalanced.

Since I'm a fan of terrible and over simplistic analogies let's say the frequency of a healthy kidney is the repetition of 1 1 1 1 1 1 1 but then I start introducing 3,s 4,s 8,s eventually the kidney will get confused and 1 1 1 1 will entrain and turn into 1 4 8 3 1 3 etc. This is the processed food, the lack of good sleep, the sugary drinks, alcohol, stress, drugs. What your job is to keep the kidney in an environment where it can be itself 1 1 1 1. Have you ever had a job or been around people where you feel like you can't be your AUTHENTIC self? It's terrible, The 1111 pattern can start to fragment and break down, before you know it you are stressed, sick, tired and not on the path or around the people you should be.

Vibrational therapy, sound healing, correct diet and nature, good friends can help us get back to all 1s so to speak.

Using various instruments paired with intention, sound healers can help to rebalance the body's systems. These instruments' vibrations and frequencies can help improve circulation and stimulate the body's natural healing processes. As our understanding of the body's energy systems continues to evolve, sound healing and vibrational therapy will likely play an increasingly important role.

In the future, we may see the development of technologies that can pinpoint the optimal frequency for each body part and introduce those frequencies to eliminate illness and disease altogether (Which I feel we have already but that's another subject).

Here are just a few noted machines that use frequency to heal already:

- Electrotherapy devices use electricity to stimulate muscles, nerves, or other tissues. Some examples include TENS (transcutaneous electrical nerve stimulation) units, often used for pain management, and EMS (electrical muscle stimulation) devices can be used for muscle rehabilitation.
- PEMF (pulsed electromagnetic field) therapy

devices: These devices use electromagnetic fields to stimulate cells and tissues in the body. PEMF therapy is often used for pain management and to improve circulation.

- Laser therapy devices use laser light to stimulate healing and reduce inflammation. Laser therapy often treats various conditions, including muscle and joint pain, wounds, and skin conditions.

- Ultrasound machines: These machines use high-frequency sound waves to produce images of the inside of the body. Ultrasound is often used for diagnostic purposes but can also be used to deliver targeted sound waves to treat certain conditions, such as muscle spasms.

The effects of vibration and sound on the body depend on the frequency, intensity, and duration of exposure. The concept of frequency is central, as all matter comprises atoms and molecules that vibrate at specific frequencies.

Whether you subscribe to the Big Bang or not, at some point, energy was converted into matter, and this matter is the foundation of the universe we know today. Atoms and molecules vibrate and oscillate at specific frequencies, and the electrons in an atom occupy particular energy levels with corresponding vibration frequencies. In sound healing, the term "frequency" typically refers to the pitch of a sound, which is measured in Hertz (cycles per second). Higher-frequency sound waves have a higher pitch and a sharper quality, while lower-frequency sound waves have a deeper pitch. By introducing the correct sound frequency, practitioners aim to help balance the body and mind.

We use music and sound for entertainment, expression, celebration, ceremony, leisure, communication, and more. Whether we are musically inclined or not, it is the one thing that genuinely connects humans from all cultures and corners of the earth.

CYMATICS

Sound healing is closely intertwined with the field of cymatics, which explores the visible patterns and effects of sound and vibration on various substances like water and sand. Vibrations and frequencies can influence the structure and patterns of liquids, which is of great significance as our bodies are predominantly made up of water, blood, and other fluids.

"The universe is not only made of particles; it's made of vibrating patterns, and cymatics offers us a glimpse into this hidden harmony."

\- Nassim Haramein

"Through cymatics, we discover that every sound carries with it a unique visual signature, a testament to the interconnectedness of all things."

\- Peter Sterling

"The study of cymatics reminds us that the boundaries between science, art, and spirituality are often blurred, and there is much we have yet to understand about the nature of reality."
- Jill Mattson

The renowned scientist Dr. Emoto conducted extensive research by photographing water crystals under a microscope and studying their structures and patterns. He claimed that the crystal structures were impacted by various factors, such as thoughts, words, and music, and that they can change in response to these influences. His book has detailed pictures of these findings.

Dr. Emoto's research suggests that how we interact with water, such as speaking kindly or aggressively, can affect its pattern and structure. This idea leads to the ongoing scientific debate about whether water can "remember" or retain information. People also debate if water itself holds consciousness. Below is a list of some of the more notable works from Dr. Emoto.

After studying cymatics I even started looking at crop circles, snowflakes etc way differently.

"The Hidden Messages in Water" (2004): This book is perhaps Dr. Emoto's most well-known work.

"The True Power of Water" (2005): In this book, Dr. Emoto further expands on his theories and

discusses the potential implications for human health.

"The Secret Life of Water" (2006): Dr. Emoto continues his exploration of water's properties and connection to human consciousness.

"The Healing Power of Water" (2007): This book delves into the potential healing properties of water and how our thoughts and emotions can affect our health.

"The Shape of Love" (2008): Dr. Emoto presents his ideas on the power of love and gratitude in this work. He discusses the concept of "Hado," which he describes as the intrinsic vibrational energy of all things.

"The Miracle of Water" (2012): Dr. Emoto explores the connection between water and consciousness.

Not only the study of cymatics, but all the elements are complex technologies. While we are taught that air is necessary for breathing, water is hydrating, food is essential, and sunlight is important, each of these are advanced technologies far beyond their surface-level explanations. Similarly, our mind, body, and cells are incredibly advanced technologies.

Personally, I would advise personal experimentation with all the elements. One that can have the biggest effect in your life is experimenting with different types of water, spring water, distilled water if you're going to remineralize it with trace minerals, structured water, having shungite or different crystals in your water, tensor rings, different water containers. Doing a fast for a few days with only water, really trying to learn these advanced technologies that we are surrounded by that are nature = Natural.

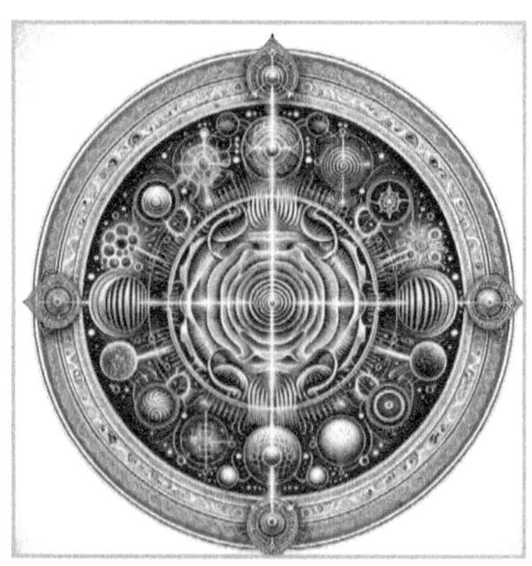

Dancing with water the new science of water by MJ pangman and Melanie Evans is a GREAT read. Their website also has tensor rings and different cradles or salts you can add to your water.

Exploring the nuances of deep breathing versus shallow breathing, nose versus mouth breathing, abdominal, rectum, chest or throat breathing, kundalini etc. Nutrition by nature, sun gazing, earthing. The possibilities for using and understanding each of these natural technologies within the natural elements can be life changing and life saving.

The deeper our understanding of these technologies, the more intentional our lives can become. By discovering our reason for being on this path and continuously learning to embody our highest version, we can help hold that space for others. This is the foundation of sound healing and most holistic practices.

INTENTION

As the saying goes, "thoughts become things." The power of intentionality is a fundamental aspect of sound healing. It's comparable to going to the gym: the more you backup your intention with action, the more likely you are to achieve your desired outcome.

When speaking of intention, I always think of the law of the triangle which is relevant in various teachings but for me it really clicked when studying rosicrucianism. The law of the triangle is based on the premise that any perfect and complete manifestation results from the union of two conditions of opposite nature. From this I developed something that I teach in sound baths called I.A.O. Intention, Action, Outcome. When you picture a triangle, it has 2 sides that come to a point forming a third. Woman + man = child, Hungry + food = full. Lots of people have lots of ideas all the time but without adding that second angle the desired result never manifests. But something still manifests; it just won't be the desired result. Your dream + Procrastination = no dream which still equals something, probably just lots of suffering and regret.

Being specific and detailed with your intentions is how to manifest them into physical reality. For instance, if you set the intention to eat well, the term "well" is WAY too vague. By contrast, if you specify what "well" means to you and create a clear action plan, achieving your goal becomes more accessible. Similarly, asking the universe for a new car requires more specific information: what kind of car, how much money does it cost, what color, for what purpose, and by when? Being particular AND SPECIFIC in which actions you will be taking increases your chances of success.

All the ancient mystery schools emphasized the importance of specificity and intentionality in manifesting one's desires. This simple concept is often overlooked.

I was at lunch one day with a friend who still battles with addiction. They were talking about wanting to get clean and that they were excited about it. I said something like "oh thats cool im happy for you, that will be good. By their body language and smile I could tell that my approval and validation made them happy and then after that they shortly changed the subject.

I listened to them for a moment but then I went back to that subject and said "okay so for you to get clean where will your daughter be staying? Are you going to do it at your house or a center? If a center, what center? How much does it cost? How long will this take? Do you need my help financially or will I need to watch your animals during this period? I told them, "I think it's good you want to get clean; we could literally just take like the next 2 hours here at lunch and plan it all out". Their enthusiasm was gone completely, they seemed irritated at the whole concept and probably rightfully so as to her I could have been coming across a certain way, maybe my tone or the fact I was actually trying to have her get specific. But at that moment I had a deeper thought.

The thought wasn't about her but it was about the overall mentality around the cycle and mindstate of poor minded people versus successful minded people, I'm not strictly speaking about finances either. I'm talking about the actual mindstate an individual carries which is usually the result of how they were raised, conditioned through media, friend groups, family and paired with their personal experience.

My conclusion is that poor minded people are usually stuck in survival mode so it's hard for them to think long term, I know this from personal experience in my past when I didn't feel like I had the time to care about whatever a 401k is when I was literally counting change just to have enough gas money to go buy my son diapers.

I don't think the poor minded person feels they have the financial and emotional freedom for the 4 hour long conversation going over each specific detail about how they are going to achieve whatever idea it is they are talking about that they could only manifest in the future when their consumed by the immediate fear of how are they even going to pay their bills today.

But that doesn't mean that they don't still have ideas so it's still nice to get the dopamine, approval and validation from vocalizing them.

Talking about it can trick your brain and make you think that you have completed it or are already there in a way even if you are currently stuck.

Think of how many people at coffee, lunch, dinners etc will tell you about some business idea or thing they are excited about or want to create. Once you get into the very specific details they either don't know them, get bored or annoyed. The difference with actual successful minded people is that these 3-4 hour extremely detailed and specific conversations is what excites and drives them. They don't care about the dopamine from ideas, they want the finished blueprint and roadmap to get it done. It's the actions that follow the intention which completes the manifestation process.

To tie this in with sound healing.

Sound healing works in dualities: receiving or sending, calming or activating, clearing or creating. Sound baths, meditation, mantras and different holistic techniques, can work and help to align you with the frequency of what you want to create and manifest. Know your why and think about why you are wanting to do sound baths in the first place ? Why during them are you having people lay down versus sitting up? Are you wanting to give a performative and theatrical sound bath with dozens of bowls or are you wanting to heal people with specific vibrations with maybe 2 bowls and a tuning fork ? What type of people do you want to work with ? 90 percent of sound baths online all look the same. But it's up to you to decide what you are wanting to use sound for ? because performing with 20 bowls on stage for 300 people is different then placing bowls full of warm water on someone's body in a one on one, versus doing a sound bath for 6 people with their eyes turned up to the ajna chakra and toning AUM.

The more specific and detailed your intentions, the easier it is to manifest them with the help of sound.

My advice to practitioners is to Allow yourself to approach sound healing with kindness, receptiveness, patience, and mindfulness. Recognize that your state of mind, and emotional well-being before you play are of greater significance than your theoretical knowledge or technical expertise. While it can be helpful to learn about music theory and frequencies, the intention behind your practice holds the most weight.

You can sense the energy of a space, person, or situation, even if you don't have a highly developed intuition. The power can be welcoming or unwelcoming, negative or positive. It may not even be directed at you but rather a projection of someone's internal state. When you really understand this, you can learn to let go of taking things personally and begin to observe and empathize with others. You can choose to see the lessons in difficult situations and recognize that life happens for you, not to you.

As sound healing and other holistic practices continue to gain popularity and become more accessible to the general public, be aware of the potential pitfalls of developing an ego or sense of entitlement around one's perceived spirituality. It's important to remain honest with oneself and to recognize that external possessions or information do not define who we are or make us better than others.

As we continue to learn and grow, we must remember that we are always students and that there is always more to learn from others. Instead of trying to convert or convince others, our role as healers and practitioners is to educate, help, and support individuals wherever they are on their personal journey.

Personally at the point of writing this I am disappointed with some of the ego and entitlement I have seen in the spiritual community especially with certain online influencers who have made a living off portraying love and light when behind the scenes they are not. It's not my place to judge and the fact I find it disappointing is my own lesson on observing why it irritates me. I spent many years in the music industry seeing things you would expect to see in the industry but then to sometimes see the same face behind a different mask in the spiritual community is unfortunate.

"Your strength as a healer is only as strong as your grace through moments of turmoil."

Its not about how you act and who you are when everything is going your way and perfect. When the lights and cameras are on, it's who you are and what you embody when it's all gone to shit. How much grace do you retain through those moments because those are most of the moments you will be expected to help others through.

Chapter 2:

EXPLORING THE PAST/ COLORING BOOK

HISTORY

The melodies of birdsong, the rhythmic crash of waves upon the shore, and the gentle rustle of leaves in the wind have always been aligned with our innate state of being.

However, as we've strayed further from nature's way, we've slowly become aware of the potential harm this deviation can bring. Cities, televisions, radios, and Wi-Fi signals have become commonplace. These frequencies can pervade our environment, and we can absorb them without realizing their impact. We no longer take the time to sit in silence or in nature, despite this being a basic human need, to help clear our minds, release, or get clear about our goals.

"Noise pollution is the most underestimated form of pollution, yet it has severe consequences on human health." - Dr. Arline L. Bronzaft, *Noise Specialist and Environmental Psychologist.*

"Noise, unwanted sound, is the most common occupational hazard in American workplaces." - National Institute for Occupational Safety and Health *(NIOSH)*

"Everything in life is vibration." - Albert Einstein

"Sound is a vibration that touches every aspect of our being." - Dr. Mitchell Gaynor, *Integrative Oncologist and Author*

The deeper you go into sound and vibration, the more you realize and notice its impact. I was watching the movie SuperMan, Man of Steel, and I saw a scene where General Zod gets his helmet knocked off or something and for the first time he has to take in all the sounds of the city, it disables him and drops him to his knees. This highlights the normalized conditions we've accepted and draws attention to the aspects of our health that we've neglected

While modern treatments and pharmaceuticals have become widely adopted, there is a growing recognition of their potential unnatural side effects. As a result, more individuals seek solace in traditional and holistic approaches to healing. These ancient practices were the first medicines.

This section will highlight factual and mythological accounts related to sound healing, significant publications, and cultural associations. We will also delve into the history of sound being utilized for healing but also as for a weapon.

Here are some gods and goddesses from various mythologies associated with sound:

Apollo (Greek mythology) - God of music, poetry, and the arts.

Pan (Greek mythology) - God of shepherds, music, and wild places, often depicted playing his pan flute.

Saraswati (Hindu mythology) - Goddess of knowledge, music, and the arts.

Odin (Norse mythology) - God of wisdom, poetry, and magic, often depicted with a harp or lyre.

Khepri (Egyptian mythology) - God of creation, rebirth, and the morning sun, often depicted as playing a tambourine.

Hathor (Egyptian mythology) - Goddess of love, beauty, and music, often depicted holding a sistrum or playing a lyre.

Apollo (Roman mythology) - God of music, prophecy, and poetry.

Orpheus (Greek mythology) - Demigod of music, poetry, and song, said to be able to charm beasts and even the gods with his music.

Kokopelli (Native American mythology) - God of fertility, agriculture, and music, often depicted playing a flute.

Oshun (Yoruba mythology) - Goddess of love, fertility, and the arts, often depicted holding a fan or playing a drum.

Ame-no-Uzume (Japanese mythology) - Goddess of dawn and mirth, often depicted dancing and playing a flute.

Krishna (Hindu mythology) - God of compassion, love, and music, often depicted playing the flute.

Thoth (Egyptian mythology) - God of writing, knowledge, and magic, often depicted playing a musical instrument and singing hymns.

Demeter (Greek mythology) - Goddess of agriculture and harvest, often associated with music and dancing.

Note that some of these gods are from mythological traditions, while others are worshiped by non-mythological religions.

Let us explore a handful of instances across different cultures where sound has been employed for therapeutic purposes.

ANCIENT GREECE

One of the earliest documented instances of sound healing can be traced back to ancient Greece. The Greeks subscribed to the belief that music could have a therapeutic impact on both the mind and the body.

The renowned philosopher Pythagoras developed the concept of the "music of the spheres," stating that celestial body movements generated cosmic music that could be utilized for healing. The pythagorean sourcebook and library by Kenneth Sylvan and David Fideler is a good read for more on this.

Hippocrates, often deemed as the Father of modern medicine, also recognized the potential of music as a tool for treating various medical conditions. He extensively wrote about the healing power of music in his celebrated medical texts. The Pythagorean school of music profoundly influenced the development of Western music theory, and many of its teachings were adopted by later philosophers and musicians.

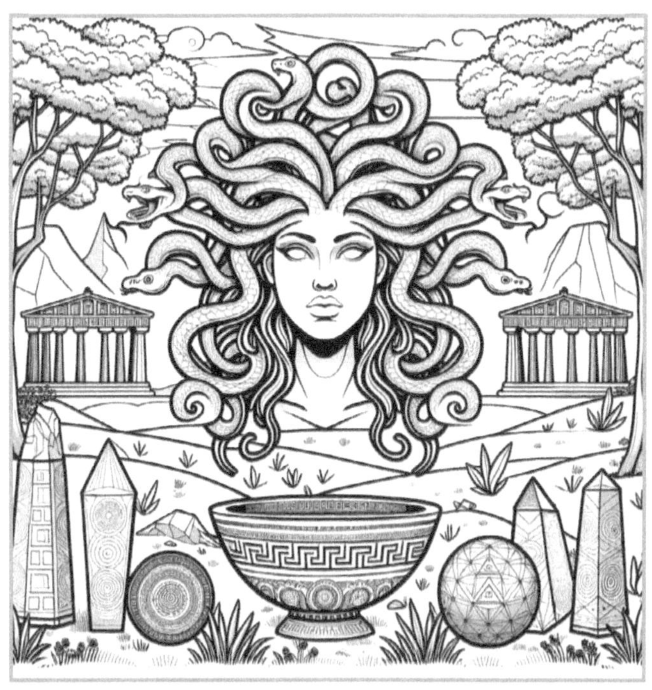

Today, the legacy of the Pythagorean school of music can be seen in the continued use of musical tuning and intervals in modern Western music. It's worth noting that the belief in balancing the four elements through music was a common idea in ancient Greece and was not unique to the Pythagorean school of thought. The ancient Greeks believed that the four elements were fundamental components of the universe and were in a constant state of balance and interaction. In Greek mythology, Apollo, the god of music. According to the legend, Apollo was a skilled musician who taught humans how to use music for healing. He reportedly employed his musical prowess to heal the sick and the wounded.

VIKING

Galdr, a form of chanting, was utilized by the Vikings for healing and protection. This practice involved reciting specific words and sounds to conjure a mystical effect. In addition to galdr, the Vikings employed drumming as another form of sound healing. Skaldic poetry, a poetic tradition used for storytelling, was also believed to have curative properties.

Viking culture is rich with myths associated with sound. According to one such myth, Odin, the god of war and wisdom, employed sound to heal wounded soldiers on the battlefield. Another legend posits that the Vikings used specialized instruments, like the Viking horn. It is widely believed that the Vikings relied on sound to cure various ailments, from physical injuries to mental disorders.

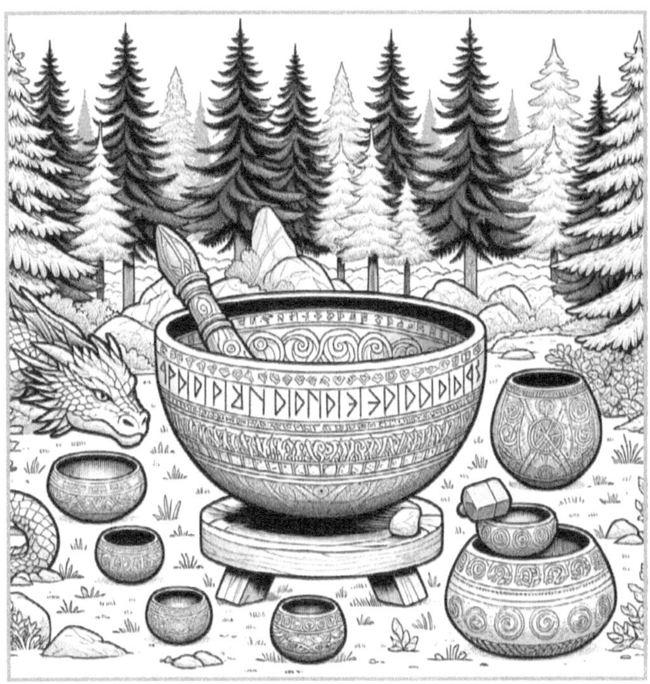

CHINA

Traditional Chinese Medicine (TCM) has a rich history of using sound to promote healing. Alongside acupressure, acupuncture, and herbal medicine, TCM practitioners have employed sound healing techniques to significant effect. Qi Gong, a form of exercise and meditation used in TCM, is a prime example. Qi Gong practitioners utilize sounds like "ahh" and "om" (Aum) to stimulate the body's energy and promote healing.

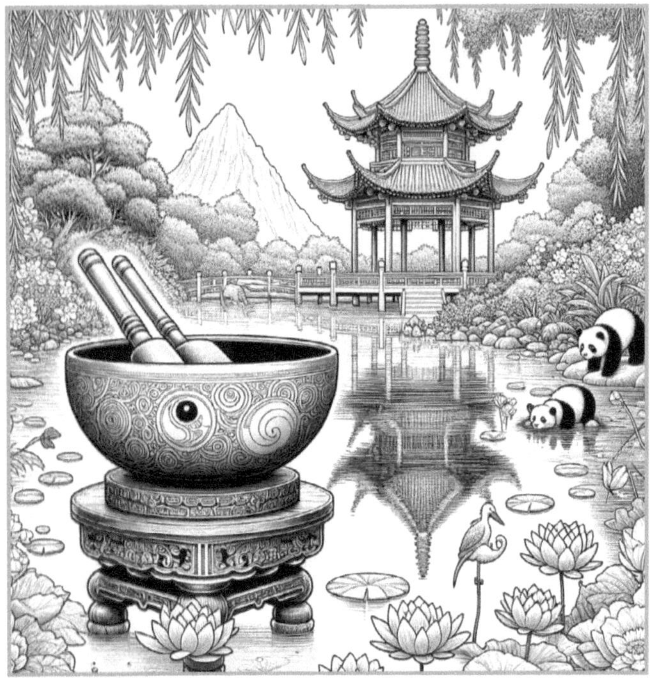

Even Chinese Opera singers were believed to possess powerful voices that could heal the body and mind. The Chinese believed that different types of sound carried various healing properties; high-pitched sounds were used to stimulate the body's energy, while low-pitched sounds promoted relaxation. Legend has it that the Yellow Emperor, a legendary figure in Chinese history used sound to heal his health problems and then taught others how to utilize sound for healing. Other tales suggest that the

Chinese used special musical instruments like the guqin and the erhu to produce healing sounds with vibrations that could penetrate deep into the meridians.

EGYPT

The ancient Egyptians deeply understood the power of sound and vibration and used different techniques to harness this power for healing and spiritual purposes. They used the sistrum, a musical instrument made of bronze or copper that produced a rattling sound, in religious ceremonies to ward off negative energies.

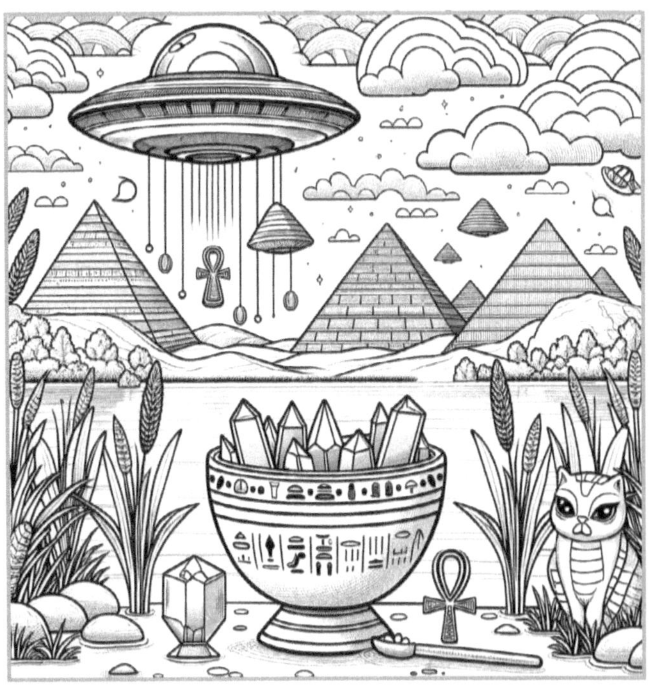

Chanting and vocal toning were also used to heal various body parts, with different sounds corresponding to other organs. Instruments such as harps, flutes, and drums were used. The pyramids, one of the most iconic structures of ancient Egypt, were believed to have been constructed using precise sound frequencies and vibrations, and some researchers suggest that they were built as suitable chambers for sound and spiritual purposes. Even certain chambers are tuned to certain hertz.

John Stuart Reid's acoustics research in the pyramids has provided strong evidence that the Egyptians designed their chapels and burial chambers to be reverberant to enhance sonic-based ceremonies.

INDIA

Ayurveda, an ancient Indian system of medicine, has long recognized the power of sound as a tool for healing. Practitioners of Ayurveda use sound therapies, including mantras, chanting, and singing bowls.

Additionally, certain forms of yoga, such as Nada Yoga, utilize sound to meditate and heal.

Indian classical music is also believed to have healing properties. According to Indian culture, one myth surrounding sound healing is that the god Shiva, known as the lord of dance and music, used sound to effect the universe and taught others to do the same.

Additionally, they are believed to have used special musical instruments like the sitar and tabla to produce healing vibrations that benefit the body.

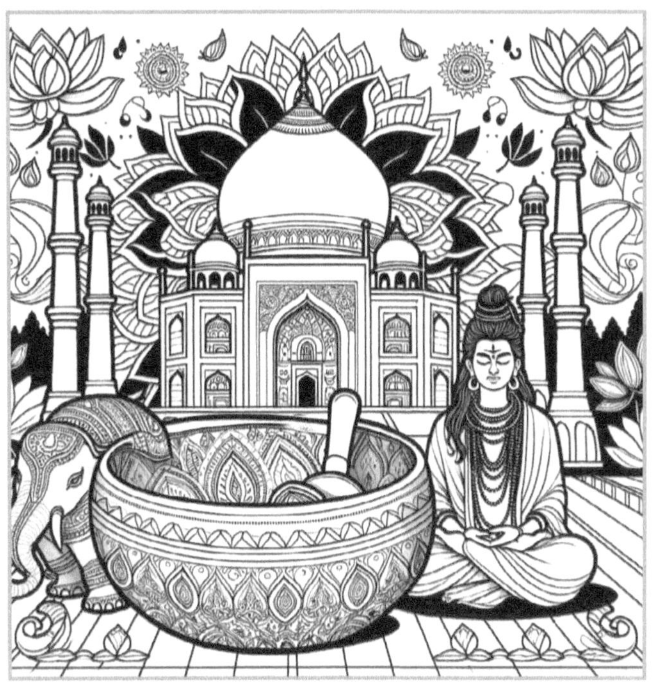

ITALY

Dating back to ancient civilizations such as the Etruscans and the Romans. During the Italian Renaissance, there was a renewed interest in the therapeutic power of music, with composers such as Giovanni Maria Artusi and Giulio Caccini creating music specifically for healing purposes.

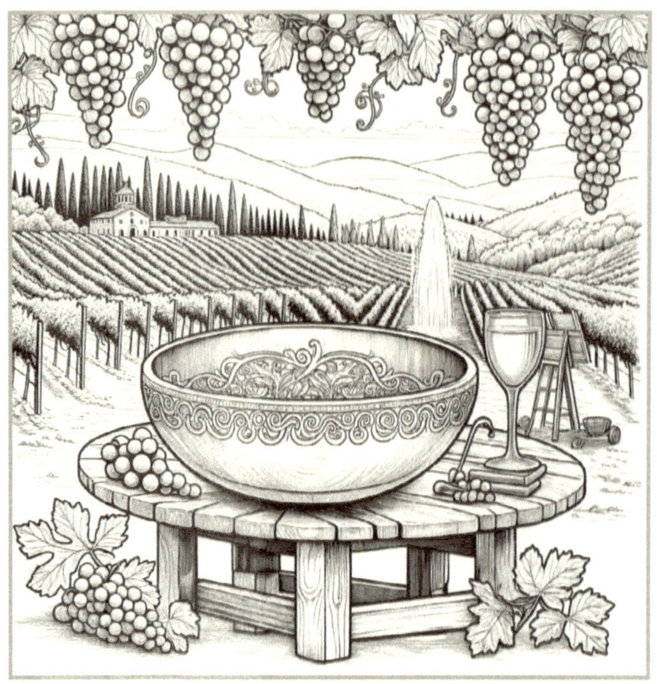

In the 20th century, Italian physician and scientist Alfred Tomatis developed the Tomatis Method. This sound therapy treats many conditions, including hearing, speech disorders and emotional difficulties. However, there is a myth in Italy that sound healing is a panacea that can cure all diseases and ailments.

AMERICA

In the early 1900s, legendary inventor and scientist Nikola Tesla explored using sound waves for therapeutic purposes, convinced that sound held the key to unlocking the universe's secrets. Later, in the 1920s, American osteopath Dr. Harold Saxton Burr developed the theory of electro-dermal activity, which suggested that the body's electrical fields could be measured and influenced by sound vibrations.

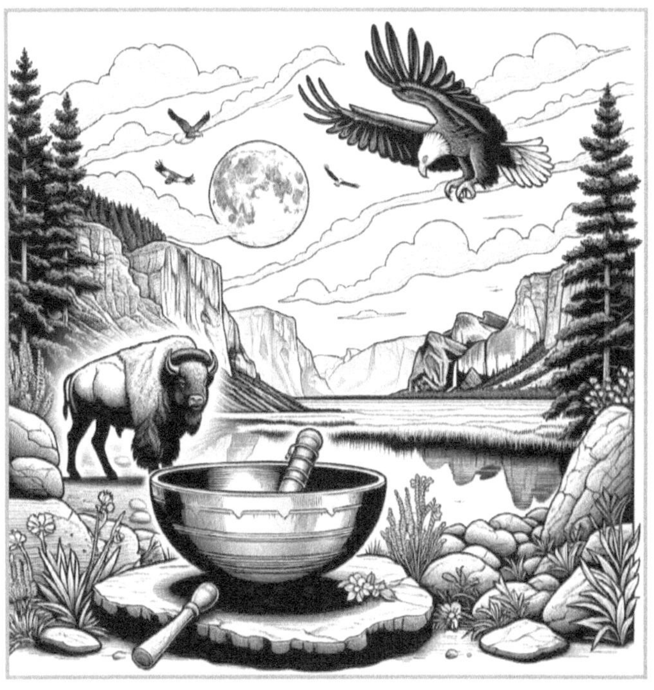

During the 1940s, the United States military incorporated music into their programs to recuperate army personnel during World War II, marking the official dawn of music therapy.

In the 1970s, musician and composer John Beaulieu created the Body Tuners, a set of tuning forks tuned to specific frequencies that could be used for sound healing.

Early publications on the therapeutic value of music appeared in the late 1700s and early 1800s, including an article in the Columbian Magazine titled "Music Physically Considered" and two medical dissertations by Edwin Atlee and Samuel Mathews.

In the 1980s, sound healer Jonathan Goldman founded the Sound Healers Association, which advocates for using sound for healing and hosts annual conferences. Dr. Mitchell Gaynor, an American author and researcher, integrated sound healing into his oncology practice and authored "The Healing Power of Sound" in 1999, which helped to popularize sound therapy in

America. Although some may view sound healing as a mystical or magical practice, many good healing techniques are based on scientific principles. They can be explained through the study of physics and biology.

AFRICA

African healing practices have long utilized chanting, drumming, and singing to create therapeutic environments. In West Africa, the kora, a 21-stringed harp, is a popular instrument used for healing, as it is believed to have the power to communicate with the spirit world. Meanwhile, the indigenous San people of South Africa employ the trance dance — a ritualistic dance accompanied by chanting and drumming.

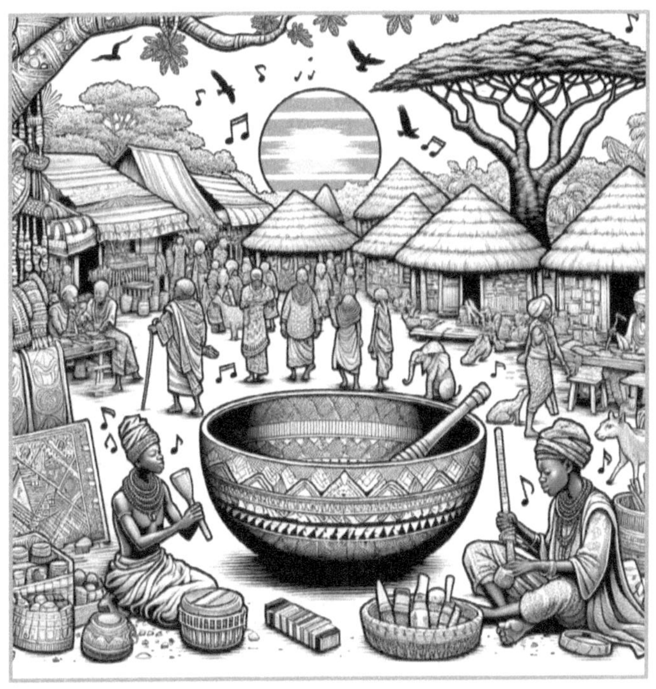

AUSTRALIA

Aboriginal music includes a range of instruments, such as didgeridoos, clapsticks, and bullroarers, which are used in ceremonies and rituals for healing and connection to the land. In modern Western approaches, sound healing is often used as a complementary therapy alongside conventional medical treatments.

Practitioners use a variety of instruments and techniques, such as crystal singing bowls, gongs, tuning forks, and voice. One of the pioneers of sound healing in

Australia is Dr. John Diamond, who worked on the concept of "toning" in the 1970s. Toning involves using the voice to create specific sounds and vibrations that can affect the body and mind. Dr. Diamond also developed the "Life Energy" concept and its connection to sound and music. Another prominent Australian sound healing community figure is Dr. David Parsons, who founded the Australian College of Sound Therapy in 2006. The college offers courses and training programs in sound healing and has developed its own method called the "Harmonic Egg." Sound healing is also used in hospitals and healthcare settings in Australia, with some hospitals offering music therapy programs for patients with conditions such as chronic pain, cancer, and dementia. The University of Melbourne offers a Master of Music Therapy program, which trains music therapists to use sound and music to improve the health and well-being of individuals and communities.

The Aboriginal people of Australia are the first known culture to heal with sound. Their 'Yidaki' (modern name, didgeridoo) has been a healing tool for at least 40,000 years. The Aborigines healed broken bones, muscle tears, and illnesses of every kind using their enigmatic musical instrument. Interestingly, the sounds emitted by the yidaki align with modern sound healing technology. It is becoming apparent that the wisdom of the ancients was based on "sound" principles.

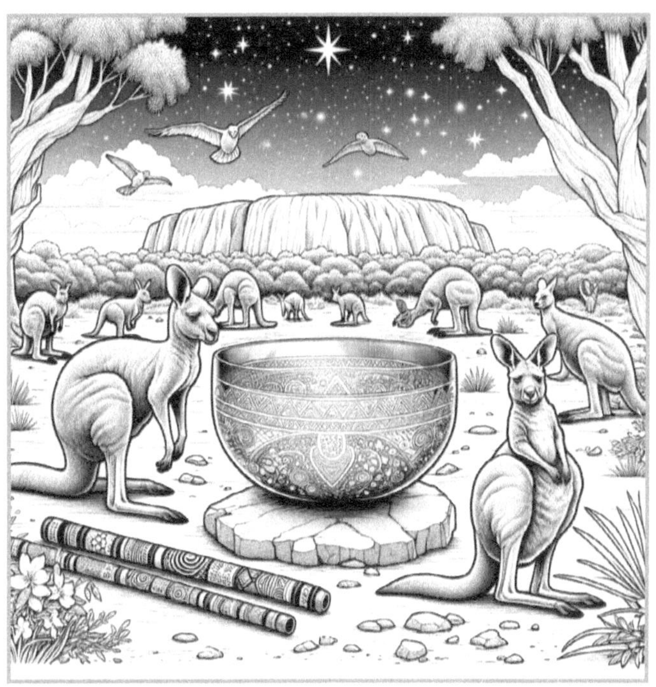

MEXICO

Known as "curanderismo" or "healing by the curandero."
Mexican sound healing practices feature instruments,
such as rattles, drums, flutes, and singing bowls, and
often incorporate singing and chanting. Some indigenous
Mexican cultures utilize sound healing to connect with
ancestors and the natural world and to communicate
with the spiritual realm. The Spanish colonization of
Mexico brought Catholicism, and with it, the use of bells
and chimes in religious ceremonies. In the 20th century,

Mexican composer and music therapist Georgina Derbez developed the "musicalization of the chakras," a sound healing technique that uses specific musical notes to balance the body's energy centers.

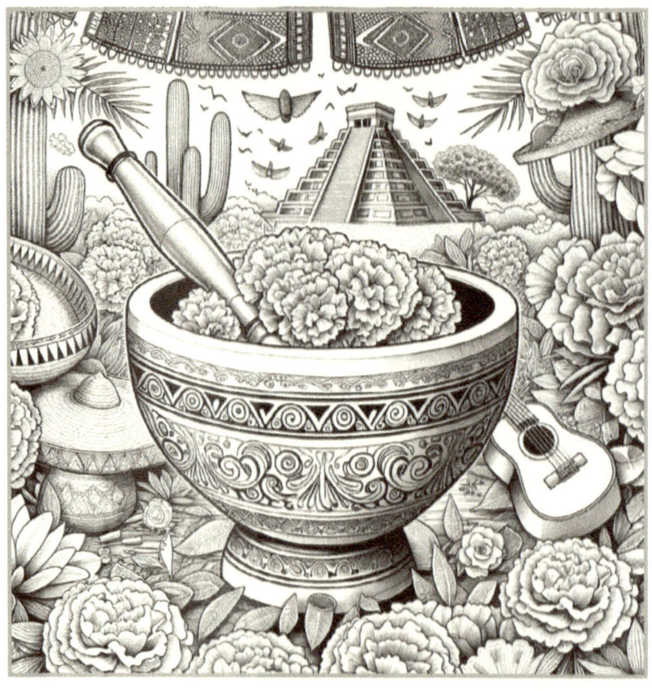

There are several common themes across cultures regarding the power of sound. Many view sound as a universal language that surpasses cultural and linguistic barriers, allowing for communication with the spiritual realm or one's inner being. This belief underscores the notion that sound possesses a profound ability to transcend physical limitations and connect us with something greater than ourselves.

OLDEST INSTRUMENT

The origins of music can be traced back to ancient times, with the oldest known musical instrument being a bone flute discovered in 2008 in Hohle Fels Cave in southwestern Germany. This remarkable find, dating back approximately 42,000 to 43,000 years ago during the Upper Paleolithic period, was crafted from the hollow wing bone of a griffon vulture and featured five finger holes.

Other ancient instruments have also been unearthed, such as the Divje Babe flute, a bone fragment from a juvenile cave bear dated approximately 43,100 to 67,000 years ago. Despite its age, this flute's authenticity remains controversial and is debated among archaeologists.

In addition to bone instruments, the oldest known lithophones, musical instruments that produce sound by striking or rubbing flat stones together, were discovered in France at an archaeological site dating back to the Middle Paleolithic period (c. 250,000 - 100,000 BC). These fascinating discoveries provide a glimpse into the earliest forms of music and the creative ingenuity of our ancient ancestors.

MODERN TIMES

In more modern times, sound and vibration are used in many fields:

Bioresonance therapy

Electromagnetic field therapy

Music therapy

Vibroacoustic therapy

The story of Dr. Royal Raymond Rife and his work with sound and vibration is fascinating. Born in 1888 and living until 1971, Dr. Rife was an American inventor and scientist whose groundbreaking work in microbiology led to the development of the "Rife machine." This device, which used radio waves to target and destroy harmful microorganisms in the body, was claimed to cure cancer and other diseases by exposing them to their specific resonance frequencies. Despite early success in treating cancer patients, Rife's work was met with skepticism from the medical community, and his claims were never "scientifically proven". Although some alternative practitioners continue to use Rife machines and other frequency-based heating modalities. Certain figures, such as Dr. Royal Raymond Rife has been associated with various conspiracy theories and claims of government cover-ups.

You can still buy rife machines and one person who I really value has an item called qi coils. I would suggest checking them out. You can find them online by searching for david wong. There are also lots of scalar and frequency based centers popping up in each town. If you are in Utah I suggest you check out Holographic Human Technology center located in Murray Utah.

The modern world of sound owes much of its development to Dr. Hans Jenny, a pioneering Swiss physician and researcher conducting groundbreaking experiments in cymatics. Dr. Jenny's research inspired the emergence of sound healing by visualizing sound vibrations on various substances like sand, water, and metal plates. His influential book, *Cymatics: A Study of Wave Phenomena and Vibration*, published in 1967, is considered one of the earliest modern texts on sound healing. Since the publication of Dr. Jenny's book, numerous other books and resources have been published, delving into specific sound healing techniques, instruments, and applications for various health conditions.

WEAPONIZED SOUND

While sound, frequency, and vibration can be used for healing, factual stories of their use as weapons exist. For instance, law enforcement agencies and military forces have used sound cannons as a non-lethal weapon to disperse crowds. Sound cannons are loud and high-pitched noises can cause pain and disorientation.

Similarly, the Long Range Acoustic Device (LRAD) emits a high-pitched, directional sound beam that can cause permanent hearing damage in those exposed to it. Military forces and law enforcement agencies have also used sound bombs, which emit a loud, high-pitched noise to disorient and incapacitate attackers or enemies.

Moreover, ultrasonic and infrasonic waves have been researched for use as non-lethal weapons. These sound waves can cause discomfort, pain, and even internal organ damage. Using sound as a weapon can have consequences, including permanent hearing damage and other health issues.

FANTASY

Now that we have delved into the history of sound, I would like to share some fascinating instances from fantasy novels where sound is used. This is for all my fellow fantasy readers out there, and as a self-proclaimed fantasy nerd, I couldn't resist.

Here are some captivating characters from fantasy novels that use sound as a tool for healing or a weapon:

Kvothe from "The Kingkiller Chronicle" by Patrick Rothfuss - Kvothe is a gifted musician who uses his singing voice and music as a potent weapon and a healing tool.

Elayne Trakand from "The Wheel of Time" series by Robert Jordan - Elayne is a powerful channeler who manipulates the elements, including sound, to heal and fight her battles.

Raistlin Majere from the "Dragonlance" series by Margaret Weis and Tracy Hickman is a skilled sorcerer who uses his magic, including sound-based somatic spells, to defeat his enemies.

Eilonwy from "The Chronicles of Prydain" by Lloyd Alexander - Eilonwy is a princess with mystical abilities, including the power to control sound, which she uses to heal others and defeat her foes.

Sympathy users from "The Name of the Wind" by Patrick Rothfuss - Sympathy is a magical system that manipulates energy, including sound waves.

Sympathy users can create devastating sound-based attacks or use sound waves for healing purposes.

These are only a few examples of fascinating characters from fantasy novels who use sound as a healing tool or a weapon.

RECOMMENDATIONS

Lastly, it's worth acknowledging the contributions of established associations that have been working on sound and healing for many years.

The American Music Therapy Association (AMTA) is the largest professional organization for music therapists in the United States, offering resources, education, and advocacy for music therapy.

The Canadian Association for Music Therapy (CAMT) is a professional association for music therapists in Canada dedicated to promoting music therapy as an effective healthcare intervention.

The British Association for Music Therapy (BAMT), a professional association for music therapists in the United Kingdom, provides training, research, and advocacy for the use of music therapy in healthcare.

The Australian Music Therapy Association (AMTA) is a professional association for music therapists in Australia, offering education, research, and advocacy for the use of music therapy in healthcare.

The World Federation of Music Therapy (WFMT) is an international organization for music therapy representing over 35 countries, promoting music therapy as a complementary healthcare intervention.

These associations not only offer valuable resources, education, and support for music therapists but also help to promote the use of music therapy as a complementary healthcare intervention worldwide.

Here is also a list of some books on sound healing that I recommend:

1. **"The Healing Power of Sound:** *Recovery from Life-Threatening Illness Using Sound, Voice, and Music"* by Mitchell L. Gaynor

2. **"The Yoga of Sound:** *Tapping the Hidden Power of Music and Chant"* by Russell Paul

3. **"The Power of Sound:** *How to Be Healthy and Productive Using Music and Sound"* by Joshua Leeds

4. **"Sound Medicine:** *The Complete Guide to Healing with Sound and the Human Voice"* by Wayne Perry

5. **"The Complete Guide to Sound Healing"** by David Gibson

6. **"Sound Healing:** *Vibrational Healing with Ohm Tuning Forks"* by Marjorie de Muynck

7. **"Tuning the Human Biofield:** *Healing with Vibrational Sound Therapy"* by Eileen Day McKusick

8. **"The 7 Secrets of Sound Healing:** *Includes 4 Free Audio Healing Downloads"* by Jonathan Goldman

9. **"Healing Sounds:** *The Power of Harmonics"* by Jonathan Goldman

10. **"Vibrational Sound Healing:** *Relaxation, Stress Reduction, and Pain Relief with Sound"* by Marysol González Sterling

11. Sarah Auster has written the book **"Sound Bath:** *Meditate, Heal, and Connect through Listening,"* which serves as a guide to incorporating sound and mindfulness practices into daily life.

12. **Crystal Singing Bowls:** *The Angelic Sound of Healing, Relaxation and Spiritual Awakening 2023* by Ashana Lobody

Chapter 3:

SINGING BOWL DIFFERENCES

MESOPOTAMIA

In the realm of online documents, a few sources claimed that Singing bowls boasted an ancient lineage spanning over 5,000 years. These documents assert that singing bowls originated in Mesopotamia.

Although the historical accuracy of this claim remains a subject of debate, I find it interesting to briefly delve into the realm of Mesopotamia, given its rich tapestry of culture, enthralling stories, captivating mythological figures, and how the musical heritage of Mesopotamia continues to influence contemporary Middle Eastern music.

Mesopotamia, often heralded as the "Cradle of Civilization," occupied a significant place in history as a region in the eastern Mediterranean. Today, it encompasses parts of modern-day Iraq, Syria, Turkey, and Iran. This historical domain holds importance as one of the earliest hubs of human civilization. Its contributions to various facets of human development.

The Sumerian civilization was one of the earliest civilizations to grace its fertile lands. Flourishing from approximately 4,500 to 1,750 BCE, the Sumerians established a sophisticated society characterized by magnificent city-states such as Uruk, Ur, and Lagash.

These urban centers stood as a testament to the Sumerians' remarkable achievements.

Foremost among their accomplishments was developing an intricate writing system known as cuneiform. This writing system employed wedge-shaped marks inscribed upon clay tablets. They documented their history, legal codes, religious practices, and other aspects of their civilization through cuneiform. This system allowed for the precise recording of musical compositions, including melodies, rhythms, and lyrics, providing valuable insights into the musical practices of ancient Mesopotamia.

BON CULTURE OF TIBET

While there are different theories about the origins of singing bowls, it is widely accepted that their true roots can be found in the ancient Bon culture of Tibet. Where actual physical bowls emerged in the Himalayan region and gradually became popular, spreading to nearby areas.

The Bon culture refers to the ancient pre-Buddhist spiritual and cultural tradition that originated in Tibet. It is one of the oldest known spiritual traditions in the region and predates the introduction of Buddhism.

The practitioners of Bon engage in various forms of meditation, divination, healing practices, and offerings to appease and seek guidance from the spiritual entities. Yes, singing bowls were used within the Bon culture of Tibet.

Throughout history, Bon has faced challenges and influences from other religious traditions, including the introduction and spread of Buddhism in Tibet. Over time, the Bon tradition has interacted with Buddhism, resulting in syncretic practices and the emergence of a distinct Bon-Buddhist tradition.

Today, the Bon culture thrives as a unique and vibrant spiritual tradition within Tibet and among Tibetan communities worldwide.

Regardless of their specific origins, it is undeniable that sound bowls have endured the test of time, captivating the hearts and minds of people across the ages.

A very detailed and in-depth website that also covers the origins is. https://singingbowlmuseum.com/pages/singing-bowl-history

ANCIENT BOWLS AND METALS

In their earliest iterations, singing bowls were fashioned from pure copper, harnessing the metal's inherent healing properties and its historical association with medicinal practices in antiquity. Copper, known for its anti-inflammatory attributes, has been attributed with the potential to alleviate symptoms associated with joint pain, arthritis, and rheumatism. Some individuals have reported finding relief and improved mobility by wearing copper jewelry or using copper-infused products. Moreover, copper has long been utilized in wound healing and is believed to facilitate tissue regeneration and collagen synthesis, pivotal processes in forming and repairing new skin.

Beyond its physical benefits, copper plays an indispensable role as an essential mineral for the proper functioning of the immune system. It actively contributes to the production of white blood cells and supports the activity of specific enzymes crucial for immune response. Maintaining adequate levels of copper is imperative for upholding a robust immune system. Additionally, copper acts as a cofactor for enzymes involved in antioxidant defense mechanisms. Neutralizing harmful free radicals within the body mitigates oxidative stress, safeguarding cellular health.

The historical connection between copper and healthy

blood circulation has been well-established. It is believed to contribute to regulating blood pressure, enhancing tissue oxygenation, and fostering cardiovascular well-being. The promotion of improved blood circulation yields a sense of overall vitality. These are just a few facets of copper's influence on human health and vitality.

Personally I had years where all I would wear is copper or crystals wrapped in copper as a conduit. Copper would always help me feel grounded. @TheWitchesForge on Instagram has some amazing copper and electro formed pieces.

While copper possesses unique tonal qualities and resonance, incorporating other metal alloys, such as bronze, revealed a broader range of harmonics and a more intricate sound profile in singing bowls. By amalgamating additional metals, these bowls produce a complex and captivating sound that holds immense value in sound healing and musical applications.

Nevertheless, copper is a relatively soft metal, susceptible to deformation and wear over time, particularly with frequent use. Care and maintenance are necessary to preserve the longevity and quality of copper singing bowls.

While singing bowls crafted exclusively from copper possess distinctive allure and historical significance, the evolution of these instruments has incorporated diverse materials and metal alloys, broadened their sonic possibilities and enhanced their appeal in music and sound healing.

Amidst the varied array of sound bowl creations, a steadfast tradition uses the seven metals: copper, tin, zinc, iron, lead, gold, and silver. These metals are believed to resonate with the energetic qualities of the chakras, contributing to the sound bowls' holistic benefits and vibrational properties. Referred to as "planetary" or "astrological" singing bowls, each bowl is linked to a celestial body, often aligned with one of the seven traditional planets known in ancient astrology: the Sun, Moon, Mercury, Venus, Mars, Jupiter, and Saturn.

A planetary singing bowl is typically crafted from a metal associated with its celestial counterpart. For instance, a Sun singing bowl may be fashioned from gold or brass, while a Moon singing bowl might incorporate silver or a silver alloy. The chosen metal resonates with the energy attributed to the corresponding planet.

Using planetary singing bowls in astrology-related pursuits has garnered a devoted following among specific individuals, practitioners, and enthusiasts who integrate sound healing and astrology into their holistic endeavors. Throughout its evolution, the construction of metal singing bowls has witnessed a material shift, with bronze emerging as the primary choice.

Crafted alloy known as "bell metal" or "singing bowl metal" has become the predominant material for these instruments. Comprising a blend of metals, predominantly copper and tin, bell metal offers enhanced strength and durability compared to pure copper. Bronze, renowned for its hardness, corrosion resistance, and ability to preserve intricate details when cast.

Bronze boasts a storied history in ancient civilizations such as Mesopotamia, Egypt, Greece and Rome where it found utility in the forging of weaponry, armor, and architectural structures.

Within musical instruments, bronze has enjoyed widespread popularity in constructing various percussion instruments, including cymbals, gongs, and bells.

Furthermore, it is a commonly employed material in producing brass instruments such as trumpets and trombones, as the copper-tin alloy contributes to the desired tonal characteristics and resonance.

Bronze stands as an alloy formed by the fusion of copper, tin, and zinc, harnessing the distinct qualities of each metal to create a harmonious fusion of strength, resonance, and durability.

Below is a fantastic read on the history as well.
https://www.theohmstore.co/blogs/our-stories/the-wild-and-fascinating-history-of-singing-bowls

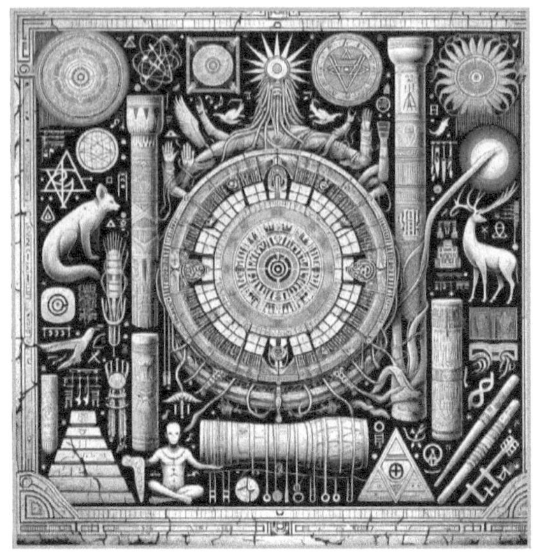

THE RISE OF THE QUARTZ BOWL

While some individuals hold beliefs that quartz and various Crystal bowls trace their origins back to Atlantis and even earlier civilizations, the theories surrounding Atlantis primarily focus on crystal, magnetism, frequency and advanced technologies, suggesting that their music and healing practices may have been based highly on vibrations, resonances and also aligned with these technologies. This has led to speculation that they might have utilized instruments similar to crystal bowls in their ancient culture. The existence of Atlantis remains a subject of debate, and there is no concrete "released" historical evidence to confirm the use of crystal bowls in that context. At least that I could find during my research.

The connection between crystal bowls and Atlantis is mainly speculative and falls into the realm of myth and ancient lore. The descriptions provided by Plato regarding Atlantis do not reference singing bowls or similar musical instruments. Plato's writings primarily focused on the political, social and philosophical aspects of the Atlantis civilization, rather than delving into specific cultural artifacts or musical traditions.

While Hermetic teachings and the writings attributed to Hermes Trismegistus discuss the concepts of vibrations and resonance, there is no direct reference to singing bowls in these ancient texts. The teachings focus on the fundamental principles of the universe, the nature of reality, and the interconnectedness of all things through vibrational energy.

The emergence of Quartz singing bowls as a distinct variation of traditional metal singing bowls in the late 20th century, particularly during the 1980s. Pioneers in this field, such as Paul Utz and William "Lupito" Jones, played significant roles in developing and popularizing crystal singing bowls. William "Lupito" Jones, the creator of the captivating Alchemy Crystal Singing Bowls (Crystal Tones®), made notable contributions to the refinement and widespread appreciation and distribution of Alchemy crystal singing bowls.

Other individuals, including Mitch Nur and various

artisans and manufacturers, have also played crucial roles in the development and widespread availability of Quartz singing bowls. Their efforts have contributed to recognizing and increasing the usage of Quartz singing bowls in sound healing, meditation practices, and spiritual pursuits.

During the 1990s and early 2000s, the popularity of crystal singing bowls experienced rapid growth alongside the rising interest in sound healing and vibrational therapies. These bowls garnered attention and were embraced by practitioners, sound therapists, and individuals seeking to incorporate sound and frequency into their holistic practices.

Quartz singing bowls are highly regarded for their ability to produce clear and pure tones, as well as their unique harmonics and sustained vibrations.

Interestingly, while there is no direct historical evidence of ancient cultures using Quartz singing bowls, a fascinating connection can be found with the computer industry. In the in pursuit of growing pure silicon chips for computers, the computer industry produced high-quality, pure silicon quartz crystal bowls. These bowls needed to meet precise standards to be recovered.

However, someone discovered their incredible pure sounds on the way to the trash bin, leading to the birth of the singing crystal bowl industry.

Since then, crystal singing bowls have become vehicles of immense potential for those working with sound. Like ancient Tibetan bowls, Quartz bowls can serve as powerful sound tools. Coupling awareness and intent in their usage can notably enhance their effectiveness.

CRYSTAL ALCHEMY BOWLS™

Referred to as Crystal Alchemy Bowls™, Alchemy bowls™ or Alchemy Crystal Singing Bowls, are a specific type of crystal singing bowl created by the company Crystal Tones® that incorporates additional elements or materials into the manufacturing process. These bowls are designed with the highest energy and intention to create unique and harmonically rich sounds and carry specific energetic properties associated with the added features and aesthetics. Alchemy bowls™ base is over 99 percent quartz with the remainder being the added ingredients, which could be anything from moldavite to rose quartz. The company had to create most of their own technology and patents to accomplish this. The crushed quartz and other ingredients have to be heated to 2600-4000 degrees, melted, molded etc.

Ive seen a little bit of the process myself and it's extremely extensive. It can take weeks for certain bowls to come into existence and not every bowl makes it. The combination of the quality of quartz, the quality of everything else that's added, the time, labor, tech it all goes into why the Alchemy bowls™ are high end and priced the way that they are.

On top of all that each bowl is unique and a 1 of 1. The company of course can create a myriad of rose quartz bowls but each one has its own frequency when it comes into existence. Music note, cent range, blemishes, hertz that give each bowl its own personality. The process and the results are truly innovative and remarkable.

Alchemy Bowls™ can also have etchings, designs, and custom pictures.

One of their notable creations is the SuperGrades™, a particular type of singing bowl that stands out from traditional alchemy bowls™. The SuperGrade Bowl™ is a testament to the innovation and craftsmanship of Crystal Tones® and human potential.

Fun fact. Moldevite, rose quartz, and Egyptian blue are the first bowls they created.

The intention behind Crystal Alchemy Bowls™ is to create instruments that combine quartz crystal's inherent qualities with the infused elements' intention and added energetic properties, on top of the relationship quartz has with us as humans. The bowls are used in sound healing, concerts, meditation and all sorts of spiritual practices.

I remember this one day, I was working at the Crystal Tones® store in Mt. Shasta when this Nomad looking lady came in barefoot, she was covered in dirt in an all natural earthy shamanistic type of way. You could tell that freedom to her meant living off the land. The perspective of homelessness is a little different in Shasta as lots of people there think the mountain is their home and lots of them are not actually poor they are just nomadic and deep in it.

I knew the bowls were healing tools but at that point I had heard them every day 50 hours a week for over a year, it doesn't matter who you are, humans will normalize their environment and can start to stop seeing the beauty in it in the same way that someone else sees it when experiencing it for the first time.

We had a 12 inch Divine Grandmother bowl right at the front on display. I asked the lady if I could play it for her. She took a couple deep breaths standing there and I started playing the bowl. After about 5 seconds she started crying. She said the bowl reminded her of her grandmother. The reason this was wild is because she didn't know that it was a grandmother bowl. It also helped me to have that remembrance and re awakening to the mission and how powerful sound can be. How everything is sound, how it does transcend language and how each of us can benefit from developing a relationship with it.

People always ask what the difference is between metal and quartz bowls.

Crystal Singing Bowls and traditional metal singing bowls differ in several aspects, including their material, sound quality, and energetic properties.

Here are some key differences:

1. ***Crystal Singing Bowls:*** Made from quartz or other crystal materials. Quartz crystal has unique piezoelectric properties, which can generate an electrical charge when subjected to pressure or vibration.

2. ***Traditional Singing Bowls:*** Made from metal alloys, such as copper, tin, or brass. The specific composition of the metal affects the bowl's sound and resonance; you can reach some lower octaves but they usually don't resonate nearly as long as Crystal Bowls.

3. ***Crystal Singing Bowls:*** Produce clear, pure tones with a long sustain. The sound is often described as ethereal, celestial, and uplifting. Crystal bowls can create a range of harmonics and overtones.

4. ***Traditional Singing Bowls:*** Generate rich, metallic sounds with a mix of fundamental tones, harmonics, and overtones. The sound can be warm and very grounding.

5. ***Crystal Singing Bowls:*** When played, crystal bowls produce strong vibrations that can be felt throughout the body. The vibrational energy is often described as penetrating and resonating deeply.

6. ***Traditional Singing Bowls:*** Also produce vibrations, but the tactile sensation can be different due to the nature of metal construction. The vibrations

are generally felt as a subtle humming or buzzing sensation.

7. ***Crystal Singing Bowls:*** Quartz crystals are associated with metaphysical and healing properties. Different crystals used in crystal singing bowls are believed to carry specific energetic qualities, enhancing the healing and vibrational effects, take emerald versus platinum for example. The quartz is also believed to resonate with humans more deeply because we have silica and quartz like compositions that run throughout our body, cells, glands etc

8. ***Traditional Singing Bowls:*** While traditional singing bowls are also considered to have therapeutic benefits, they are not inherently linked to specific crystal energies, we also don't have the same abundance of metals inside of us that we do with quartz and our crystalline structure .

9. ***Crystal Singing Bowls:*** Manufactured by shaping and molding pure quartz crystal using specialized techniques. The process involves heating and cooling the crystal to create a precise tone and resonance.

10. ***Traditional Singing Bowls:*** Handcrafted through hammering and shaping metal alloys, resulting in a unique shape and design. The craftsmanship and techniques used by skilled artisans contribute to the bowl's sound quality.

These factors contribute to the distinct characteristics and experiences of crystal and traditional singing bowls, making them suitable for different purposes and personal preferences within sound healing and spiritual practices.

SUPER GRADES™

If you have personally heard one of these then you already know the power behind them and if you have never heard one I suggest that you seek and then relish the opportunity as soon as you get it.

Here are some benefits for Crystal Tones® SuperGrade Bowls™:

They offer exceptional qualities that set them apart from standard bowls.

100% Pure Crystal Quartz: Supergrade bowls™ are crafted using 100% pure ethically sourced crystal quartz, as other Crystal Bowls are 99% plus, give or take. This ensures the highest level of purity and clarity in the bowl's composition, allowing for pristine sound resonance and vibrational qualities.

Unique Technology: Supergrade bowls™ incorporate special technology and innovative manufacturing techniques. These advancements in bowl construction enhance the bowl's overall quality, durability, and resonance. The result is a superior sound healing tool that offers an unparalleled experience.

Extremely Rare: Supergrade bowls™ are exceptionally rare, with less than 1% of the world having the opportunity to experience them in person. Their scarcity adds to their exclusivity, making them highly sought after by sound healers, practitioners, and enthusiasts.

Increased Quartz Content: Supergrade bowls™ can contain approximately 10 times more quartz material than standard bowls. This increased quartz content accelerates and amplifies the bowl's intention and vibration, allowing for a more robust and transformative sound healing experience.

Resonance: Supergrade bowls™ produce a resonance that sets them apart. When played, they can sustain their vibrations for extended periods without external stimulation. This extended resonance adds depth and richness to the sound, creating a truly immersive and captivating sonic experience.

Supergrade bowls™ represent the epitome of luxury and excellence in crystal singing bowls. With their pure quartz composition, ethical sourcing, advanced technology, rarity, amplified intention, and luxurious resonance, they offer sound healers and enthusiasts an unparalleled tool for achieving profound healing, relaxation, and transformation.

When you hear a supergrade it can literally be life changing. You feel the vibrations coming off the bowl and it penetrates through your entire being. The 14-16 inch super grades will resonate for 5-10 minutes on their own as you will feel and still hear the low pitch rumble. I've watched light workers feel fully charged after playing these for 5 min and i've watched addicts start to literally sweat and detox within 10 min of playing these. They are extremely powerful healing tools that have been brought into creation.

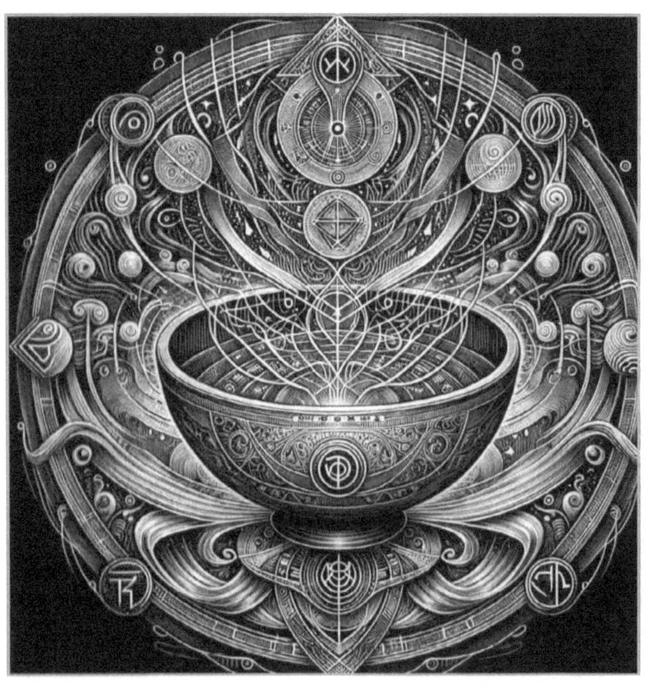

Chapter 5

ENERGY CENTERS

CHAKRAS

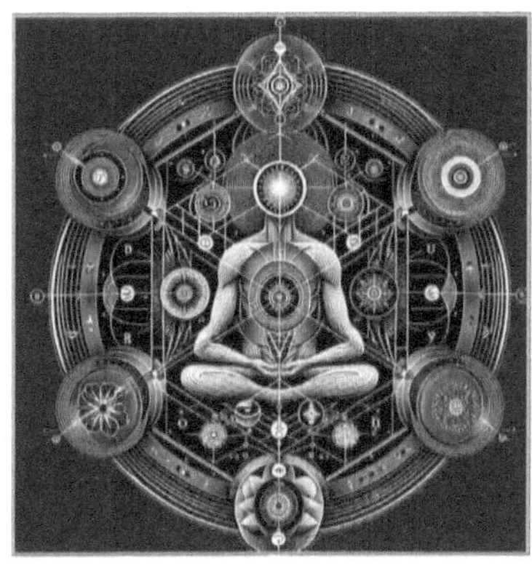

The concept of chakras has become popular among individuals seeking holistic healing and self-improvement. Many books, blogs, and websites have touched on these for quite some time. Rather than attempting to reinvent the wheel, this chapter will concentrate on the connection between chakras and sound healing, particularly with Singing bowls. This piece will provide an overview of their significance for those unfamiliar with chakras. Additionally, tips and tricks will be provided to identify possible chakra imbalances in others. Finally, some simple yet effective techniques will be explored to enhance one's practice.

"The body is held together by sound. The presence of disease indicates that some sounds have gone out of tune." - Deepak Chopra

Chakras are energy centers in our body that help us feel healthy and balanced.

Everything from gut issues to the way we speak come from either balance or imbalance within the body. According to the teachings of the spiritual teacher Sri Guru Amit Ray, it is believed that there exist 114 chakras, but we are only going to be addressing the primary. According to a variety of research on chakras, You have seven energetic wheels inside your body going up your spine, and each wheel has a different energy of what it is responsible for. Each chakra represents a different body part and different things you feel, like happiness, love, lust, rage and so on.

Traditional Indian and Hindu texts, where the concept of chakras originates, did not initially ascribe specific colors to them. The modern color system for chakras is believed to have been popularized and standardized by Theosophists and other Western esoteric thinkers in the late 19th and early 20th centuries.

Your mind, body and spirit all feel aligned and healthy when all the energy centers within yourself are in harmony. When they are not you can feel sick, tired, overly excited, or another range of emotions and health conditions can manifest. So, eating healthy foods, getting enough sleep and exercise, positive affirmations, not being consumed by stress and continuing to do things that sit well with your nervous system is key. In key, in tune, in harmony. Ask yourself what is the soundtrack that you have created for your life, what is the song that you are playing today. What do you want to be the reflection of ?

BRIEF HISTORY

The word "chakra" originates from Sanskrit and means "wheel" or "mystical energy circles." The term is closely linked to the yoga traditions of Hinduism, which view chakras as vital centers of energy within the body. Originating from the yoga traditions of Hinduism, the word "chakra" holds great significance in this ancient religion's spiritual and philosophical practices. It is said that the human body contains 114 chakras and 72,000 nadis, which represent divine energy and the network of energy flow. Early Sanskrit texts describe chakras as meditative visualizations combining flowers, mantras, and physical entities within the body.

However, the seven main chakras that run along the spine are the most widely known and studied among modern-day practitioners.

Kundalini yoga, techniques in specific breathing exercises, visualizations, mudras, bandhas, toning, chanting, kriyas, Sound baths, and Color therapy are focused on manipulating the flow of subtle energy through the chakras. Leading to a simple state of peace and divinity within oneself to achieve states of higher consciousness and spiritual enlightenment.

The main text about chakras that have come to the West is a translation by the Englishman Arthur Avalon (Sir John George Woodroffe) in his book, The Serpent Power, published in 1919. Since then, hundreds of publications, events, workshops, etc., have been around the chakra system.

SINGING BOWLS

Singing bowls in relation to sound healing have gained immense popularity as people seek alternative forms of therapy to improve their health. In this context, chakras often come up in conversations related to sound healing and singing bowls.

Each layer of the sound healing plays into its overall effect on the body, mind and spirit. Sound healers, students, teachers, and practitioners who work with singing bowls can often focus on specific areas of the body or energy centers, known as chakras.

Using their intention when playing the bowls, they can direct the healing vibrations towards particular energy centers.

Understanding the chakra system is beneficial for anyone working with sound healing and singing bowls. Moreover, knowledge of the chakra system can be helpful when working with individuals who are experiencing specific issues in their lives. People may not be familiar with chakras but may still describe specific physical or energetic imbalances in their bodies. In such cases, practitioners can use their knowledge of the system to identify the possible underlying causes of inequality and direct their sound healing techniques.

One of the most common things people tend to question when it comes to the chakras is whether they are real. Regardless of whether one believes in their existence, there are more than likely still aspects of their life that they could work on or improve upon. Whether it be personal relationships or physical ailments, the chakras offer a unique perspective on addressing these issues.

Now, let's elaborate on the chakra system with singing bowls.

The music notes listed on the singing bowls reflect the seven primary energy centers and integrate five critical components of the endocrine system. Additionally, a thirteenth element is incorporated to symbolize wholeness and completion. This intricate design is inspired by the chromatic music scale and its alignment with the chakras, where each note corresponds to a specific energy center.

It is not uncommon for individuals unfamiliar with energy work or other holistic concepts to feel overwhelmed by the complexity of such topics. This is where breaking down the chakra system simplistically can prove helpful.

Let's start from the bottom of the chakra system and work our way up.

ROOT CHAKRA

- Muladhara (root chakra) Mula' means root and Source, and 'dhara' means foundation
- Music note, C
- Color, Red
- Element, Earth
- Mantra, "LAM"- I Am
- Stones, Stones: Red Jasper, Brown Jasper, Hematite, Smoky quartz, Cuprite, Mahogany, Obsidian, Tourmaline, Rhodonite, Bloodstone, Garnet
- Physical Properties. Base of spine, perineum, legs, feet, skeletal system, colon, bladder, kidneys.
- Energetic properties.

Feeling grounded, stability, security, safety, connection to Earth, and ancestry.

The root chakra is a component of the human body's energy system, representing the foundation upon which all other chakras build. Positioned at the base of the spine and connected with the color red, this chakra is also known as the Muladhara chakra.

Imagine being stranded on a deserted island, completely stripped of all possessions. No clothes, no tools to build shelter or gather food, no money, no place to even spend it. You are left with nothing but your mind and body and the dwindling daylight hours before darkness descends.

Forcing you to confront the raw essence of your being and test your will to survive, this is where the root chakra comes into play.

Our innate drive to secure our basic needs—shelter, sustenance, stability, security, and safety—is an instinctual response from the Root Chakra. This energy center is our rooting in the world and grants us the grounding energy that enables us to connect with our physical existence and navigate the challenges that accompany it. Through the root chakra, we can form a relationship with the Earth, ourselves and the natural world, this helps us to get real about our situation and how to navigate it.

Suppose that our need for security, stability and safety still needs to be met. In that case, we may experience anxiety, fear, jealousy, insecurity, stubbornness, lack mentality and become disconnected and cut off from our potential blessings.

The significance of the Root Chakra's influence extends beyond the stranded island scenario, as its impact remains relevant to the aspects of our daily lives that bring us stability, security, and a sense of foundation.

In contemporary times, this pertains to our professional pursuits, job security, financial security, housing arrangements, feeling secure in our relationships, and having trust in those situations, which all play a vital role in maintaining our sense of stability and balance.

The Root Chakra is like the foundation of a house: if it's shaky, everything else is bound to come crashing down. When this chakra is out of balance, you might also experience physical symptoms like lower back pain, sciatica, digestive issues, restless legs, feet issues and constipation. Your emotional state can feel like a total rollercoaster, leaving you feeling like you're floating in a sea of uncertainty.

Some people may also have an overabundance of energy in the root chakra, which can manifest as a being entitled, self centered, ego driven, or inflexible attitude towards change. By maintaining balance in this energy center, we can experience a sense of security, stability, safety, and connection.

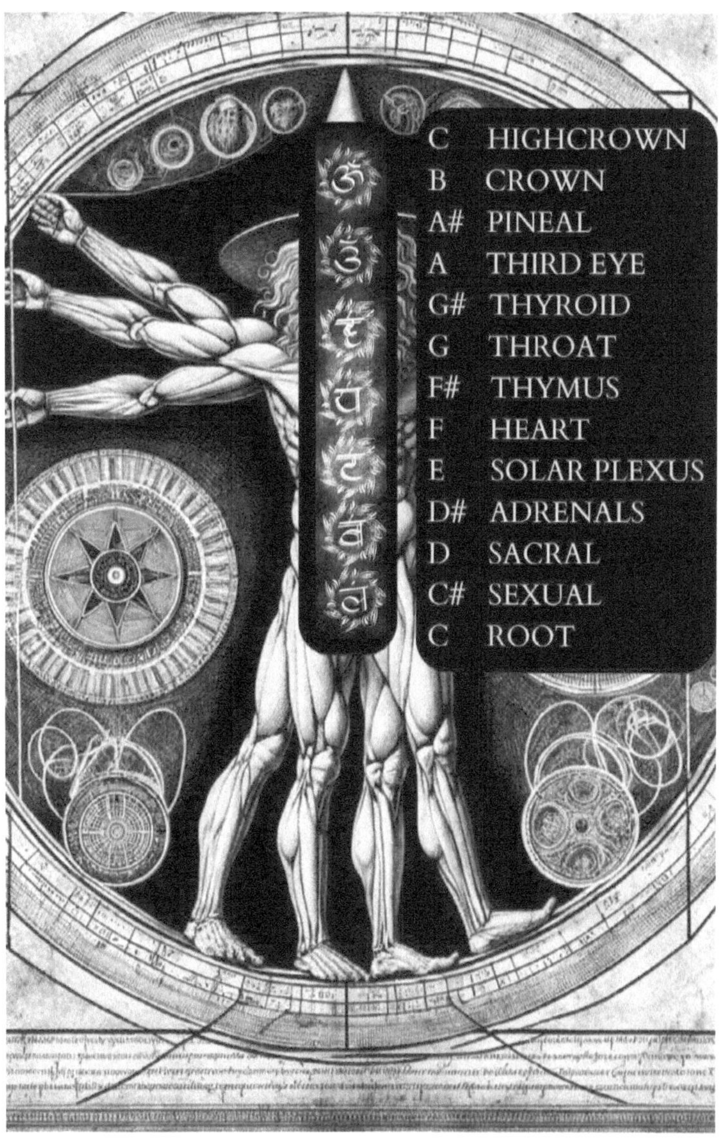

C   HIGHCROWN
B   CROWN
A#   PINEAL
A   THIRD EYE
G#   THYROID
G   THROAT
F#   THYMUS
F   HEART
E   SOLAR PLEXUS
D#   ADRENALS
D   SACRAL
C#   SEXUAL
C   ROOT

SACRAL CHAKRA

- Svadhisthana (sacral chakra)
- Music note, D
- Color: Orange
- Element, Water
- Mantra, "VAM"- I Feel
- Stones, Stones: Carnelian, Obsidian, Unakite, Orange calcite, Red Jasper, Sunstone, Citrine
- Physical Properties. Lower abdomen, hips, lower back, reproductive organs, prostate, sacrum and womb
- Energetic properties. Creativity, artistry, sexuality, intimacy, emotions, emotional processing, and being in flow.

The sacral chakra, the second of the seven primary energy centers in the human body, is called the Svadhisthana chakra. Positioned in the lower abdomen, precisely beneath the navel, this chakra is typically characterized by the vibrant color of orange.

The sacral chakra is a powerful center of energy within the body, intimately connected with our emotions, creativity, and relationships. When this chakra functions harmoniously, we experience a sense of freedom and vitality that allows us to fully express ourselves, Create, and connect deeply with others.

Imagine for a moment that you worked on your root chakra and that your root chakra is well-balanced and taken care of. You have a strong foundation in the world, your finances are stable, your relationships are healthy and fulfilling.

With this sense of security and grounding, you can explore new avenues of creativity and self-expression. You may find yourself building a cozy hammock in your backyard or creating beautiful works of art, exploring the idea of starting your own business.

You are more attuned to your emotional state, able to process your feelings, and connect more deeply with your loved ones. You feel comfortable with your sexuality and experience joy and intimacy.

However, when the sacral chakra is blocked or imbalanced, we may struggle with emotional instability. Our creativity may be stifled, and we may have difficulty expressing our emotions. Sexual dysfunction, such as a lack of desire or problem connecting with our partners, can signify sacral chakra imbalance.

Physically, this chakra is associated with the reproductive organs, kidneys, bladder, and lower back, and imbalances can manifest as issues such as menstrual irregularities, urinary tract infections, lower back pain, etc.

It's important to note that both the root and sacral chakras play significant roles in our lives, and when one is out of balance, it can profoundly impact the other. For example, we may encounter incredibly creative and free-spirited individuals who struggle with stability in their personal or professional lives. Conversely, someone highly successful and grounded in the material world may also be too rigid and stubborn and struggle with emotional expression and intimacy.

By understanding the role of the sacral chakra in our lives and working to balance this center of energy, we can learn to find pleasure and fulfillment in healthier ways without relying on addictive behaviors, hedonism, dopamine drivers, gambling, overeating, or other harmful coping mechanisms.

SOLAR PLEXUS CHAKRA

- Manipura (navel chakra/Solar plexus)
- Music note, E
- Color: Yellow
- Element, Fire
- Mantra, "RAM"-I Do
- Stones, Stones: Amber, Citrine, Calcite, Tiger eye, Yellow Topaz, Agate, Yellow Jasper, Yellow Tourmaline, Lemon Quartz, Sunstone
- Physical Properties. Digestive system, stomach, liver, gallbladder, pancreas, and small intestine.

Skin and parts of the nervous system.

- Energetic properties. Self-esteem, confidence, values, willpower, drive, ambition. Opinions and instincts.

The solar plexus chakra, also known as the third chakra or the Manipura chakra, is one of the seven main energy centers in the body. It is located in the upper abdomen, just above the navel, and is associated with yellow.

The solar plexus chakra embodies our inner fire, drive, and personal values. It's the spark that ignites our passion and propels us towards our goals. As we progress from the root and sacral chakras, we step into the solar plexus, where we discover our true ambition and determination.

The realization that it's not just about achieving success by following a routine or habit. It's about unleashing our creativity, standing up for ourselves, and channeling our personal power to make a difference in the world. We've all encountered people with immense creativity but need more drive to pursue it. Conversely, there are people who possess unbridled ambition but no creativity. The solar plexus chakra is the mediator, balancing these two traits. When our solar plexus chakra is balanced and healthy, we feel empowered, confident, and self-assured. We possess a strong sense of identity and willpower, enabling us to confidently overcome obstacles and pursue our dreams.

In contrast, an imbalanced or blocked solar plexus chakra can lead to feelings of low self-esteem, laziness, lack of confidence, and an inability to take action. It may even manifest as physical symptoms such as digestive issues, stomach problems, and adrenal fatigue. We must tap into our inner strength and personal power to nurture our solar plexus chakra.

We can do this by setting clear goals and intentions, acting towards those goals, and cultivating a positive self-image. Practicing self-care, asserting our boundaries, mindfulness and meditation to foster inner peace and confidence are also essential. Even setting small goals and completing them will help slowly start to develop confidence. Many people today struggle with confusion, laziness, and a lack of ambition and values, making it difficult to establish healthy boundaries and express themselves honestly.

HEART CHAKRA

- Anahata (heart chakra)
- Music note, F
- Color, Green
- Element, Air
- Mantra, "YAM"- I Love
- Stones: Rose Quartz, Green Aventurine, Emerald, Rhodonite, Green Jade, Amazonite, Malachite, Prehnite, Rhodochrosite, Green Tourmaline, Chrysoprase, Green Calcite, Kunzite, Green Moldavite, Moss Agate, Peridot
- Physical Properties. Heart, lungs, circulatory system, blood pressure
- Energetic properties. Love, compassion, empathy, and connection with others

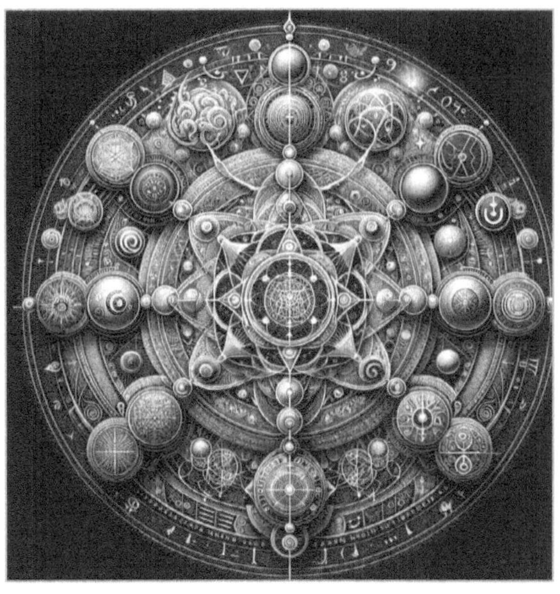

The heart chakra, also known as Anahata in Sanskrit, is the fourth chakra located at the center of the chest. It is considered the center of love, compassion, and emotional balance. The heart chakra is a beautiful energy center that radiates love and compassion. Its element is air, associated with the color green, representing growth and renewal.

However, the heart chakra is not limited to just one color, as some associate pink with this energy center. Pink is a softer, more nurturing energy that can be helpful in opening and balancing the heart chakra. When our heart chakra is balanced and open, we can experience deep egocentric and meaningful connections with others.

We feel a sense of joy, peace, and contentment in our

lives and relationships; we are able to give and receive love freely and openly. The heart chakra encourages us to cultivate self-love and self-acceptance, reminding us that it is equally important to love and accept ourselves as it is to love and give to others. Unfortunately, specific life experiences or personality traits may make individuals more prone to heart chakra imbalances. For example, those who have experienced significant emotional trauma, such as childhood abuse, neglect, domestic violence, etc., may struggle with opening their heart chakra and trusting others.

They might even have a hard time trusting themselves and their own decision-making. Feeling like choices they have made only led to betrayal or self-betrayal.

Similarly, individuals who tend to put up emotional walls, avoid vulnerability, or suppress emotions may also have a closed heart chakra. Physical symptoms associated with an imbalanced heart chakra may include heart or lung problems, high blood pressure, or poor circulation. If you are experiencing these symptoms, practicing self-care, connecting with others, attending holistic events, therapy and engaging in activities that promote emotional healing can go a long way. You get to choose the perspective and lesson from each event in your life. People who have an open heart chakra usually see such events as tools and lessons even if they are unfortunate versus taking everything personally and feeling like the world is out to destroy them.

By becoming the reflection of the world we wish to see, we inspire others to do the same. In this journey of self-discovery and self-trust, it's important to remember that what is meant for us will always find us. We don't need to force situations or chase after what isn't meant to be. We can trust that the universe has a plan for us and that everything in our lives ultimately leads us toward our highest good if we keep a clear intention and are willing to meet it halfway. When preparation meets opportunity.

THROAT CHAKRA

- Vishuddha (throat chakra)
- Music note, G
- Color, Blue
- Element, Ether or akasha, which represents space, sound, and vibration
- Mantra, "HAM"- I speak
- Stones: Aquamarine, Amazonite, Lapis Lazuli, Sodalite, Angelite, Blue Lace Agate, Blue Apatite, Chrysocolla, Blue Chalcedony, Blue Kyanite, Azurite, Larimar, Blue Calcite, Celestite
- Physical Properties. Throat, larynx, vocal chord, cervical vertebrae, esophagus, tongue, gums, teeth and ears.
- Energetic properties. communication, expression, listening, authenticity, integrity, and being able to speak up and articulate for yourself and others.

The throat chakra, also known as the Vishuddha chakra, is located in the throat area and is associated with the color blue. Its element is ether or sound, and it is responsible for our communication and self-expression. The throat chakra is a vital energy center that governs our ability to express ourselves fully and communicate effectively.

In my experience working with people, I have found that approximately 75-80 percent of individuals I encounter struggle with throat chakra issues. In today's society, we are bombarded with expectations and pressures from all directions, making it increasingly challenging to vocalize our thoughts and emotions. Social media comparison and the illusion of endless opportunities can leave us feeling lost and unsure of our true desires, let alone how to vocalize them. The throat chakra is the natural progression through the chakra system, following the root, sacral, solar plexus, and heart. It is the gateway to authentic expression, where we leave our ego behind and embody love and empathy.

A closed or imbalanced throat chakra can leave us feeling too shy, insecure, or afraid to speak our minds or be honest with others about how we think or what we want.

It is worth contemplating how many issues could have been prevented if they had been addressed on a smaller scale. For instance, when a partner chooses to make a statement like "You always do this," instead of addressing the matter the first time, It becomes a lot harder to address and unpack.

When we do speak, there can be the added difficulty of feeling unheard, judged, gaslit and misunderstood, leading to frustration and disconnection.

Repressed and unvocalized emotions or a fear of confrontation can result in energy blockages, which can eventually manifest as physical symptoms such as sore throat, hoarseness, jaw tension, neck stiffness, throat infections, teeth grinding, ear aches, and thyroid issues, to name a few and that just physical let alone the emotional damage it can cause.

Engaging in activities that promote self-expression and communication is helpful to balance the throat chakra. This can include actively speaking up for ourselves, toning, practicing active listening, and communicating with a partner, friends, family members, or places of employment. Pursuing creative outlets such as writing or singing and public speaking. Remember, nonverbal communication and body language are equally important aspects of effective communication. By prioritizing self-expression and communication, we can open up the throat chakra and achieve greater clarity, confidence, and authenticity in our interactions with others.

THIRD EYE CHAKRA

- Ajna (third eye chakra)
- Music note: A
- Color, Indigo
- Element, light, ether, space
- Mantra, "OM" or "AUM" – I see
- Stones: Amethyst, Labradorite, Lapis Lazuli, Azurite, Sodalite, Citrine, Black Obsidian, Lolite, Clear Quartz, Moonstone, Lepidolite, Purple Fluorite, Black Tourmaline, Turquoise, Kyanite

Also known as the Ajna chakra, it is situated right in the center of the forehead, nestled between the eyebrows. It is associated with the color indigo and the element of light.

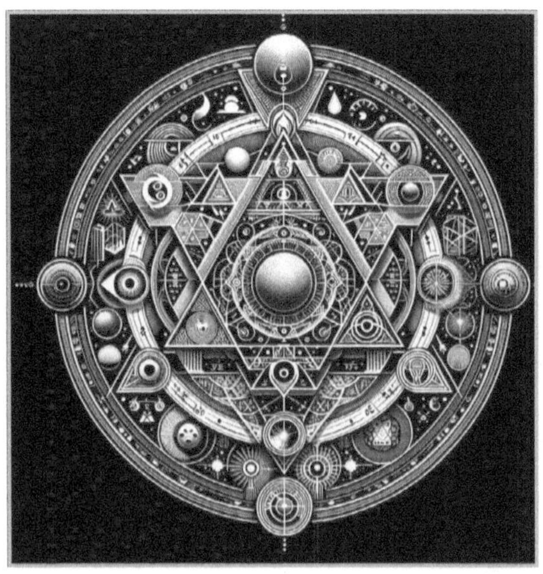

This chakra governs our intuition, wisdom, and spiritual insight.

When we speak of intuition, we refer to that inner voice that guides us in the right direction. The voice tells us what feels right or wrong, even when our rational minds cannot comprehend it. The third eye chakra amplifies this inner voice and allows us to quickly trust our instincts. Think about how many situations we wouldn't have gotten ourselves into if we trusted our intuition. How many opportunities could we have taken advantage of if we listened to it?

It helps us connect with our higher selves and tap into a realm beyond the physical, allowing us to gain spiritual awareness and insight into our lives. As we progress through the other chakras, we slowly gain a sense of confidence, trust and insight into our lives. We develop aspects of emotional mastery, enabling us to drive ourselves forward and speak up for what we believe in.

With a balanced third eye chakra, we are no longer trapped by self limiting beliefs or negative thoughts. Instead, we can see our lives clearly and understand the different paths we could take to achieve our goals.

This clarity of vision and purpose allows us to create timelines and shift our thoughts into tangible actions that bring us closer to our desires. However, when the third eye chakra is blocked or imbalanced, we may feel lost, confused, and disconnected from our future, path, and inner selves.

Our intuition may be clouded, and we may need help to trust our instincts or confidently make decisions. Physical symptoms such as headaches, eye strain, sinus, and vision problems may also manifest. This is a sign that our third eye chakra is not functioning at its optimum level, and we must take steps to balance it.

One way to balance the third eye chakra is through meditation and mindfulness researching things that help to decalcify the pineal gland. Tuning forks, sound and Energy healing is another effective way to balance the third eye chakra, with techniques such as Reiki or crystal healing being highly beneficial. Diet is a big one.

We must also pay attention to our inner voice, journal our dreams, and journal our thoughts and feelings. Within us lies a voice guiding us toward our better selves, nudging us to make choices in our best interest. However, more often than not, we choose to ignore this voice and succumb to our lower impulses.

> *"I count him braver who overcomes his desires than he who conquers his enemies; for the hardest victory is over self."*
>
> – Aristotle

CROWN CHAKRA

- Sahasrara (crown chakra)

- Music note, B

- Color, Violet or White

- Element, element of consciousness, which is often considered to be a non-physical element. Unlike the other six chakras, which are associated with one of the traditional five elements (Earth, water, fire, air, and ether), the crown chakra is believed to transcend the physical realm and connect to the divine or spiritual realm.

- Mantra, the crown chakra, is often associated with the sound of silence, representing a state of pure consciousness and unity with the divine.

- Stones: Clear quartz, <u>Amethyst</u>, <u>Selenite</u> Lepidolite, Sugilite, <u>Labradorite</u>, White Agate, <u>Lapis</u> <u>Lazuli</u>, <u>Fluorite</u>, Charoite, Moonstone, White Calcite

- Physical Properties. Metaphysical concept that refers to a center of consciousness and spiritual awareness located at the top of the head

- Energetic properties. Enlightenment, higher consciousness, inner peace.

The crown chakra, the Sahasrara chakra, is the seventh and highest chakra in the human body's chakra system. It is located at the top of the head and is associated with the color violet or white and the element of thought or consciousness. The crown chakra is the center of spiritual connection and divine consciousness. This chakra is often depicted as a lotus flower with a thousand petals, symbolizing its vast and infinite nature.

When this chakra is fully activated, it's like a portal to a higher realm of existence that opens up, allowing us to experience a sense of unity and interconnectedness with all things. What this would look like is if you ever met someone who is passionate and connected but also very unbothered. How unbothered by certain things this individual is might annoy others who are not on this frequency as this can be mis-labeled as not invested, or "they don't care" The truth is that they care deeply about everything but they also see this world for what it is.

When your crown chakra is balanced and open, you may feel a sense of inner peace. You may feel a deep connection to the universe and experience a sense of Oneness with everything around you. You are not bitter and resentful.

You may also experience a heightened sense of spirituality and a deeper understanding of the universe and your place within it. On the other hand, when the crown chakra is blocked or imbalanced, you may experience a sense of disconnection from the universe and a lack of purpose or meaning in life.

You may need help finding direction or clarity in your life and any connection to any spiritual concepts.

You can see this when someone is not open to anything not even spiritual but anything potentially even positive, it could be as simple as telling someone that lemon water is good for them and they would rebuttal by saying its witchcraft or something. Physical symptoms such as headaches or migraines may also manifest.

Reflecting on the chakra system, one can discern the significance of the crown chakra in the preceding steps. After establishing a solid foundation through the root chakra, creating emotional awareness through the sacral chakra, forming a sense of drive and values through the solar plexus chakra, developing love and empathy through the heart chakra, and honing the power of communication through the throat chakra, one can start to envision and manifest their reality through the third eye chakra.

This progressive journey through the chakras ultimately leads to the opening of the crown chakra, marking the culmination of spiritual ascension. Self-sabotaging tendencies or addiction to low-impulse behaviors can hinder one's progress. Nonetheless, with INTENTION and persistence, one can continue to ascend toward higher levels of consciousness and self-realization.

Here are some commonly used frequencies for each energy center.

Chakra Frequencies

Root Chakra
(Muladhara): 256 Hz

Sacral Chakra
(Svadhisthana):288 Hz

Solar Plexus Chakra
(Manipura): 320 Hz

Heart Chakra
(Anahata): 341 Hz

Throat Chakra
(Vishuddha): 384 Hz

Third Eye Chakra
(Ajna): 426 Hz

Crown Chakra
(Sahasrara): 480 Hz or higher

When performing a Sound healing session with Alchemy bowls™ where you are trying to clear chakras, A simple and effective way is during the session you have the person picture that energy center. For example if it's the root Chakra you have them picture the imbalances, whether that is instability in, relationships, jobs, finances, housing. Or If it's a root physical issue, As you are playing, have them breathe light and positivity into that situation, have them accept where they are at, don't avoid it as people will try to make excuses for their situation or blame others, have them take responsibility and then let all of that go, the judgment, confusion, resentment etc have them take accountability. Then have them picture what it would look like fixed and if they were living the best version of this reality that they could. Have them picture it being real already, have them get specific. What does that reality look like for them? Each breath placing more intention and affirmation into it. You can also tone in those frequencies into the person's area of the body where they are having issues. I will release more detailed and specific meditations and guides in the future.

But Here is another one to help you get started.

Chakra Cleansing and Purification Exercise

Duration: 5-10 minutes (adjustable to individual preferences)

Equipment: One singing bowl, preferably a hand practitioner or alchemy bowl around 9 inches, not too heavy for extended holding.

Instructions for Facilitator:

Prepare the Participant:
- Guide the participant to choose a comfortable position: laying down, sitting up in a chair, or standing.

Initiate Movement:

- Instruct them to start with movement:
- Wiggle and move their feet for 10 seconds.
- Progress to their knees, hips, stomach, arms, and head, moving from the root to the crown.
- Encourage a light full-body shake for 10 - 30 seconds to release tension and promote energy flow.

Short Breath Session:

- Guide the participant through a short breath session:
- Inhale through the nose for 6 seconds, deep into the stomach.
- Exhale out through the mouth for 12 seconds. Modify for shallow breathers (3 seconds inhale, 6 seconds exhale).
- Instruct them to visualize light, love, purity, etc., during inhales, capturing stagnant energy. Release on exhales, letting go of self-limiting beliefs.
- Repeat this process five times then Encourage normal breathing, making all inhales and exhales through the nose, if possible.

Chime the Bowl:

- Take control of the singing bowl:
- Lightly chime the bowl from the root to the crown

(7 chimes), taking a few seconds between each.

- If they are laying down, go from the left side up to the crown, then down the right side. If standing or in a chair, move from the front to behind, activating each chakra.

Playing the Bowl at the Root:

- Hold the bowl at the root.
- If you are new or hesitant, play the bowl with good intentions.
- Focus on health, stability, and finances, specific to each chakra.
- Play for as long as desired (30 seconds to your preference).
- Allow a moment of silence before moving up.

Optional Vocal Expression:

- If you are comfortable, vocalize the root chakra sound "LAM" or guide a meditation on abundance related to the root, such as finances and safety.

Move Up and Repeat:

- Progress to each chakra, letting moments of silence follow playing.
- After reaching the crown and playing till silence. Then start playing again, circling the person clearing anything that might be stuck in their

auric field and helping to patch any holes, before bringing the bowl directly into the heart. Have them hug the bowl and embrace it as they would a helping friend, loving family member.

Guardian.

Closing the Session:

- Conclude the session with a moment of silence.
- Keep in your mind and heart as the facilitator that the intention is to activate, clear, and purify with light and positive source energy.

Endocrine System

Now, let's talk about the Endocrine system as it applies to sound healing and Alchemy Bowls™. An easy way to explain this would be that

Our body makes a large amount of chemicals that help us do different things like grow, sleep, feel happy, or even control how fast our heartbeats. The endocrine system is what makes these hormones. It comprises different parts of our body, like the thyroid gland, the adrenal gland, and the pancreas. Each piece of the endocrine system makes other hormones with unique jobs.

Think of the hormones as messengers that tell your body what to do. They travel through your bloodstream to reach different parts of your body and ensure everything is working just right.

Without the endocrine system, our body wouldn't be able to function.

Hypothalamus,

Pituitary gland,

Thyroid,

Parathyroid,

Adrenal glands,

Pancreas,

Ovaries,

Testes,

Thymus,

Gastrolienal,

Pineal,

Kidneys,

Heart,

Adipose tissue

Each of these glands secrete hormones that regulate various bodily functions, such as growth and development, metabolism, reproduction, and stress response.

According to the American Thyroid Association, it is estimated that about 20 million Americans have some form of thyroid disease, which is only one type of endocrine disorder. Diabetes, another type of endocrine disorder in 2023, affects over 37 million Americans. Other endocrine diseases such as adrenal insufficiency,

Cushing's syndrome, and polycystic ovary syndrome also involve many people.

Alchemy bowls™ and sound healing can help facilitate healing for these systems With different bowls having a different focus also with the base of your intention. The notes on the bowls that are specific to these are.

C# Reproductive glands

D# Adrenal glands

F# Thymus gland

G# Thyroid gland

A# Pineal gland

The Reproductive Glands
(ovaries and testes) C#

Reproduction and the production of hormones that are essential for the development and maintenance of our bodies. In females, the ovaries produce eggs that can be fertilized by sperm from males, leading to the development of a fetus. In males, the testes produce sperm that can fertilize a female's egg. Both organs also have hormones such as estrogen and testosterone in many bodily processes, including growth, metabolism, and sexual development. When the ovaries or testes don't function properly, it can lead to infertility, hormonal imbalances, low testosterone, and other health problems.

The Adrenal Glands D#

These glands sit right on top of your kidneys and play a role in keeping you healthy and happy. They produce hormones that help your body deal with stress. Your adrenal glands release hormones like adrenaline and cortisol to help you cope with stress.

But what happens when your adrenal glands stop working? Unfortunately, that can cause severe problems. People with adrenal insufficiency, or Addison's disease, don't produce enough hormones. This can lead to fatigue, muscle weakness, weight loss, and even shock in severe cases. We live in a fast-paced world. We get stuck overusing them, and our bodies can only sometimes keep up with the demands we place on them. When constantly stressed out, our adrenal glands must work overtime to produce enough hormones. Over time, this can wear them out and cause them to stop functioning correctly. Another factor is our diet. Many Americans eat a diet high in sugar, processed foods, and unhealthy fats. This can lead to inflammation in the body, damaging the adrenal glands and making them less effective. If left untreated, adrenal insufficiency can lead to a potentially life-threatening condition called an adrenal crisis.

An adrenal crisis can cause symptoms such as severe vomiting, abdominal pain, dehydration, low blood pressure, and loss of consciousness. The good news is that there are things you can do to support your adrenal glands and keep them functioning well. Eating a healthy diet, getting enough sleep, and managing stress through activities like yoga, sound baths, and meditation can all help.

The Thymus gland is a small chest organ just behind the breastbone. It plays a crucial role in the immune system, particularly in developing T cells, which help the body fight infections and diseases. Unfortunately, the thymus gland can stop working correctly due to a variety of factors, including aging, specific medical treatments, and autoimmune disorders. When this happens, the immune system can become compromised. The thymus gland is the seat of our immune system, so when it stops working, it makes it harder for the body to fight off infections and diseases. You can do several things to help support the thymus gland. One should eat a balanced diet

. You can also incorporate immune-boosting foods like garlic, ginger, and turmeric. Regular exercise can also help support the thymus gland, as can getting enough rest and managing stress.

Additionally, certain supplements like vitamin D, vitamin C, and zinc may be beneficial in supporting the immune system and the thymus gland specifically.

Thyroid Gland G#

The thyroid gland is a tiny but mighty gland located in your neck. This gland produces hormones that significantly affect your body's metabolism. Metabolism is like your body's engine; it determines how much energy you burn and how fast. If your metabolism is running slow, you might feel tired and sluggish, but you might feel more energized if it's running fast. Unfortunately, a lot of people experience issues with their thyroid gland. One of the most common issues is an underactive thyroid, also known as hypothyroidism. This means that your thyroid gland isn't producing enough hormones, which can cause symptoms like fatigue, weight gain, and cold intolerance.

Once again, one major factor is stress. In today's fast-paced world, it's easy to feel stressed out all the time, which can take a toll on your thyroid. Another factor again is diet. Certain nutrients, like iodine and selenium, are important for thyroid function. If you're not getting enough of these nutrients in your diet, your thyroid gland might not be able to function properly. Remember to take breaks and do things that make you happy to help manage stress.

"Self-care is giving the world the best of you, instead of what's left of you."
- Katie Reed

The Pineal Gland A#

Or the "third eye," is a small endocrine gland deep within the brain. Despite its small size, it plays a role in regulating various bodily functions and influencing our perception of the world. The production of the hormone melatonin is at the heart of the pineal gland's function.

Melatonin is a critical in regulating the sleep-wake cycle, helping us to fall asleep and stay asleep throughout the night. It also helps to control other bodily functions such as blood pressure, immune system function, and the release of certain reproductive hormones.

However, the pineal gland's influence extends beyond just regulating bodily functions. It is also believed to play a role in our perception of the world around us, particularly in consciousness and spirituality. In various spiritual and esoteric traditions, the pineal gland is a gateway to higher states of consciousness, allowing us to connect with the divine and access spiritual insights and experiences. Furthermore, the pineal gland is also associated with producing the psychedelic compound DMT, which is believed to play a role in spiritual experiences and altered states of consciousness. The release of DMT is thought to be connected to near-death backgrounds and experiences induced by psychedelic substances such as ayahuasca.

High Crown

Lastly, there is the High Crown, which is not technically part of the endocrine system or the physical chakra system but is often included in depicting chakras, such as in the Crystal Tones® image in our booklet.

The first question that may arise is regarding the function of the High Crown and its differences from the Crown Chakra. While both are associated with spiritual development and connection to the divine, the Crown Chakra focuses on personal and physical connection to the sacred. In contrast, the High Crown is associated with one's higher purpose and soul's connection to the cosmos.

The second question may pertain to the significance of a C bowl as both a Root Bowl and a High Crown Bowl. The Root Bowl is associated with grounding, rooting, and physical connection to the Earth, whereas the High Crown Bowl is associated with a spiritual connection to the cosmos. The paradoxical use of C in both cases represents the unity, coming full circle, and interconnectedness of all physical and spiritual things. It's also the representation of completing an octave in music theory envision the chakra system as a circular journey starting from the Root (C) and progressing through each chakra until the circle is completed. This circle represents the wholeness and completion of one's transformation through the chakras.

It's not uncommon to see people seeking crystals,

sound baths, and other practices that aim to connect them to the divine, guardian angels, Ets, ascended masters, etc. While this is entirely understandable and can be a beautiful part of one's spiritual path, it's important to remember that spirituality can sometimes become a form of escapism, even another addiction.

As humans, we often seek ways to leave our bodies and escape our problems, but actual growth and healing come from finding moments of bliss, acceptance, and deep connection within ourselves.

I would ask yourself, Are you using these practices to truly achieve that or are you using them as a distraction?

People can search for anything to fill the void. Recognizing that avoiding our problems doesn't make them disappear. In fact, they may continue to manifest throughout our lives until we are forced to confront them head-on.

For example, if we find ourselves repeatedly experiencing the same issues in our relationships, it may be time to take a step back and consider whether we are the common denominator in these situations.

PRECAUTIONS

This next part serves as a precaution.

With the accessibility of information and resources, it is easy to become involved in energy, spiritual, and metaphysical practices without considering the precautions people took in the past. Every action we take in life has a reaction; this is especially true in the realm of energy work. The kybalion is a good read to understand this deeper.

Let us consider playing with an Ouija board. If a demon or malevolent spirit were to show up, would the person playing with the board know how to get rid of it ? Are they educated and prepared to handle the situation they have provoked? Do they have the tools, spells, faith, energy, mindset, and knowledge to deal with it? Similarly, there are stories of people having spontaneous spiritual awakenings that profoundly transform their lives. Stories of people who get in a car or similar accident, cross over, come back, and have a fantastic testimony, but their relationships, food preferences, career choices, everything can change during this transformation process.

Like butterflies and snakes leaving behind dead parts of themselves, individuals may also leave behind aspects of their old lives. The movie The Matrix provides an example of this, as the character Neo undergoes a significant transformation after being introduced to the concept of reality as a simulation. Keep in mind that even though these concepts are accessible to anyone nowadays, we must still consider the precautions and preparations that have been in place in the past for energy, spiritual, and metaphysical work.

Chapter 6:

SOUNDS OF THEORY

INTRODUCTION

Music is a language not just heard but deeply felt in one's being.

Music theory is the set of rules and guidelines that musicians use to make sense of that language and how music functions, how we can communicate with each other about music, and be able to play together and create new music.

This chapter aims to provide a simple yet comprehensive explanation of music theory related to Singing bowls. While the intricacies of music theory can be complex, a simple understanding can significantly enhance the effectiveness of our experience.

To begin, let's define music theory. Music theory is the study of the principles and practices of music. It encompasses everything from the fundamentals of music notation and rhythm to the complexities of composition and musical analysis. The three main elements that music consists of are Frequency (notes/pitches), Dynamics (volume), and Time (rhythm). All these three can be combined in various ways and give out different aural results, pleasant or not, and set a different mood.

At its core, music theory helps us understand music's structure and organization. One key concept in music theory is harmony.

Harmony refers to the combination of different frequencies (notes/pitches) that are pleasing (or not) to the human ear. When we combine two or more Alchemy Bowls™, we create a simple or more complex harmony. To create a pleasantly harmonious set of bowls, it helps to understand some basic musical concepts such as notes, scales, octaves, keys, and chords, just to name a few. Think of every interaction you have with someone, it's either harmonious and leaves you feeling good or there is tension, discomfort and it's disharmonious.

FREQUENCIES AND NOTES

Each sound we hear is a wave with a specific frequency in which that sound wave vibrates through the air. In music, we refer to the sound waves and frequencies as notes. After years of music evolution and history, some guidelines about how notes function together arose.

In Western Music, the octave(C4toC5) is divided into 12 steps, which are the 12 keys in the piano within an octave. To complete the octave, add the 13th key, as seen in the image below.

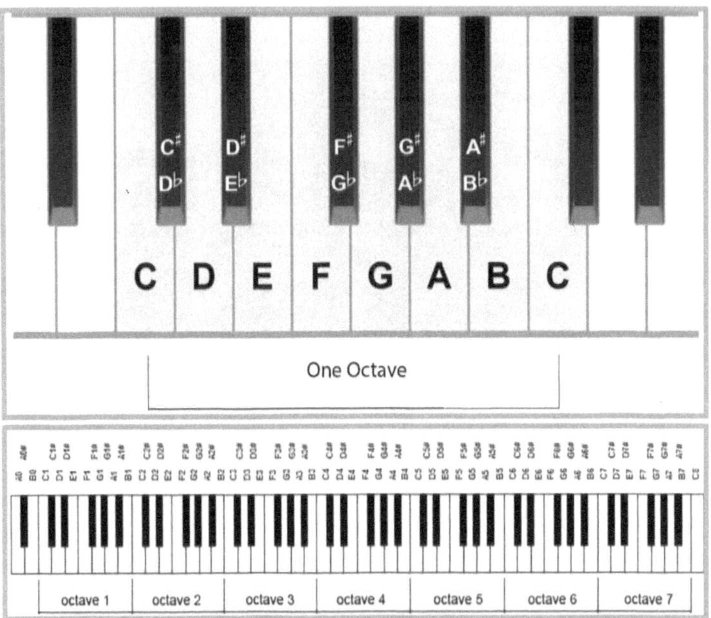

As you can see above, a standard 88 key piano has seven octaves. Most humans can only hear a total of ten octaves, and most Singing bowls more or less range from the third to the fifth octave, which currently puts most of the bowls within the 200-600 hertz range. You can also see the octave from C to C being demonstrated in the Crystal Tones® chakra sheet.

You can see in the image that 12 different notes are starting low from C all the way up and completing the octave with high C. Starting from C being the root and working its way higher up the body is similar to on a piano; when you begin at C and work your way across the piano, the notes and frequency for each letter become higher in pitch.

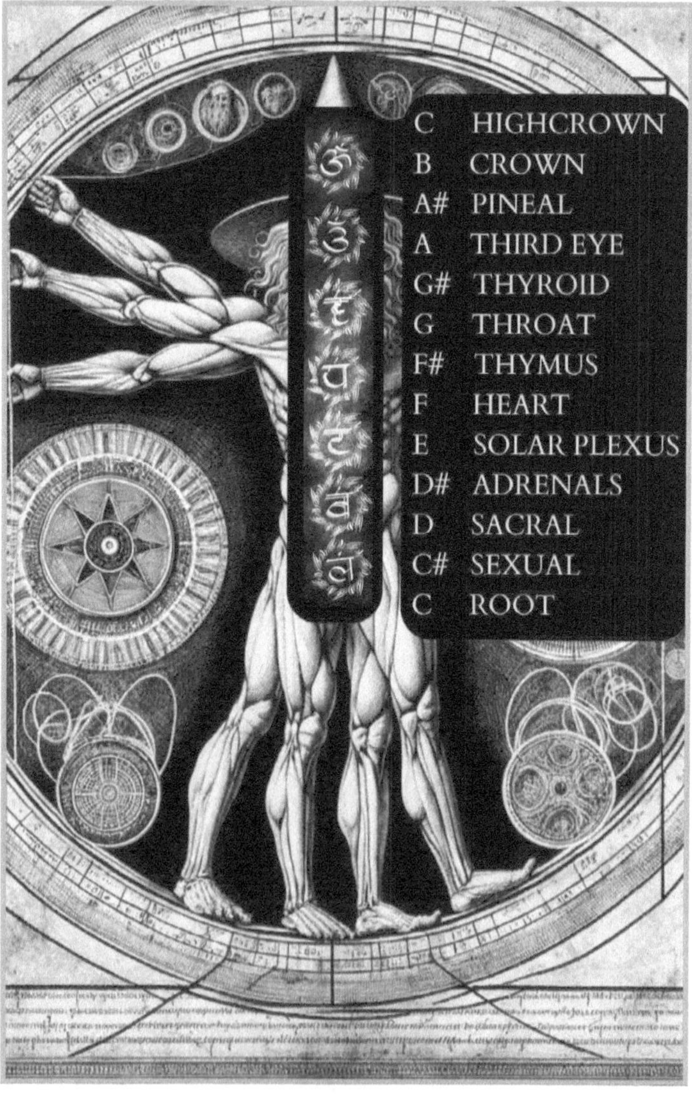

I will include another sheet below with every hertz for every note regarding equal temperament tuning (True Tone) (A440), which is what Most Singing bowls tune their bowls around.

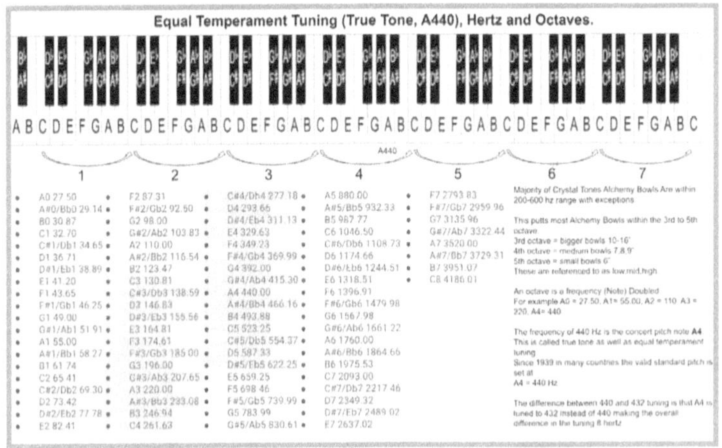

By the time the standard 88-key piano was developed in the 19th century, it was already firmly established that the first seven letters of the alphabet (A, B, C, D, E, F, G) would be used to represent the natural notes within an octave. The reason for starting on C instead of A is primarily due to the musical scale's convenience and the keyboard layout's historical evolution.

When you look at a piano keyboard, you'll notice that there are groups of two black keys followed by groups of three black keys, repeating across the keyboard.The note C is strategically placed before the group of two black keys, which makes it easy to identify. This pattern helps musicians locate notes quickly, even without looking at the keyboard. In contrast, starting on A would break the pattern and make reading and navigating the keyboard less intuitive. While alternative keyboard layouts and tuning systems are created on A, the C-centric design has become the standard for modern pianos, making them widely accessible and consistent for musicians worldwide.

SHARPS AND FLATS

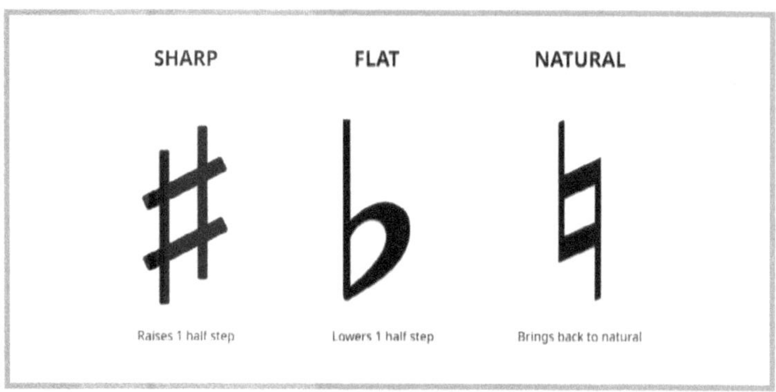

You will usually encounter three signs in music: the sharp, the flat, and the natural. As you can see, above are the natural white keys; the black keys are labeled as a sharp (#) or a flat

(b). On Most singing bowls the bowls will also be labeled with a sharp if they are sharp, it's normal to never see bowls labeled as flats. Let's take a look at what each of these signs means.

A sharp is applied to a note and sharpens it, which

means it raises it by one half-step or semitone. For example, playing an F note on the piano is on a white key. If you put a sharp next to the note F, then it's played on a black key, which is a half-step higher. A flat does precisely the opposite of a sharp one. It is applied to a note and flattens it, aka lowers it, one half-step or semitone. For example, if you play an E on the piano, it's on the white key. If you flatten it by a half-step, you will play it on the black key immediately lower than E.

To help simplify, sharps and flats tell us which notes to play in a song based on the chosen scale. A sharp arrow is like an arrow that points up, making a note sound higher. On the other hand, a flat is like an arrow pointing down, making a note sound lower. We use sharps and flats when we want to change the sound of a note. Sometimes, when we play music, we need to use notes that are not part of the natural notes in a song. Sharps and flats help us to achieve this.

SCALES

A scale is a series of musical notes arranged following a specific pattern of whole and half steps. Think of a scale kind of like ingredients you need to create a specific song. The most used scales in Western music that you may have heard of are the major and minor scales and the Pentatonic Scale in Pop, Rock, Blues, and Country culture. Each type of scale follows a certain whole-step and half-step pattern. The pattern for the diatonic Major Scale which is what most chakra sets will follow is W-W-H-W-W-W-H, and the pattern for the natural minor Scale is W-H-W-W-H-W-W. The Major and minor scales form the basis for many melodies, harmonies, and chord progressions in Western music. In the key of C major, for example, the notes of the diatonic scale follow this pattern, starting from C: C (whole step to D) D (whole step to E) E (half step to F) F (whole step to G) G (whole step to A) A (whole step to B) B (half step back to C) This pattern can be applied to any starting note, and it will produce a diatonic scale in that key. Until you retain these patterns the easiest way to to create a harmonious set of bowls would be to pick the Alchemy bowl you want then based off its note you could reference my set building chapter to see all the scales and notes that could potentially sound good with the bowl you picked.

Most Singing bowls labeling system is based on the chromatic scale (the diatonic scale we just mentioned can be created within the framework of the chromatic scale), The chromatic scale is a musical scale that includes all twelve notes, that is, the black and white keys on a piano keyboard.

The chromatic scale includes all the natural notes C, D, E, F, G, and A, as well as all the sharp and flat notes C#

or Db, D# or Eb, F# or Gb, G# or Ab and A# or Bb. Crystal Tones® uses the Chromatic scale for its framework, so these are the notes you will see on the majority of singing bowls, which we are primarily focused on. You will see all the Natural notes and the sharps on the bowls but not the flats.

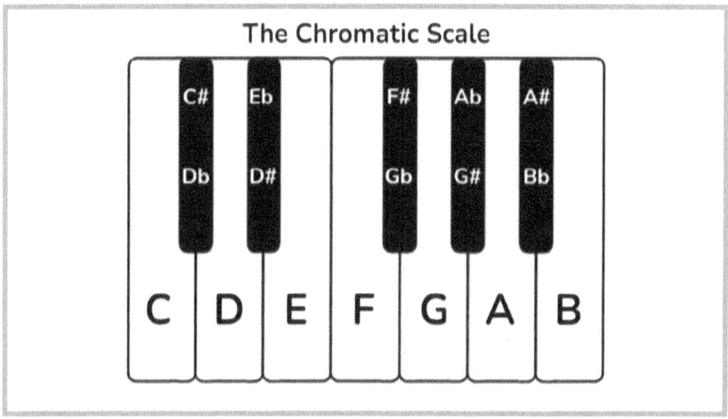

Each note has a specific pitch, which is determined by its Frequency. There are many music scales worldwide, each following its structure and format. The most common scales in Western Music, as we have said, are the Major and the Minor Scale. The most accessible scale to play is the C Major scale, and its notes are:

<u>CDEFGAB</u>

The C major scale uses only the white keys on Bb piano, so if you start on the note C and go across to the right, playing each white key in order, you'll be playing the C

Major scale. The key of C major is also frequently used as a starting point for learning music theory and how to play major scales on musical instruments such as the piano, the guitar, the violin, and so on. Depending on your instrument, many beginner-level songs and exercises are written in the key of C major due to its simplicity. To sum up the pattern or the major, here are a few examples of well-known songs that have been written in C major:

"Let It Be"by the Beatles

"Happy Birthday to You"(traditional)

"Imagine"by JohnLennon

"All of Me" by John Legend

"Twinkle, Twinkle, Little Star" (traditional)

"Für Elise" by Ludwig van Beethoven

"Hallelujah" by Leonard Cohen and

"Piano Man" by Billy Joel

"My Heart Will Go On" by Celine Dion and

"Moon River" by Henry Mancini.

"Ode to Joy" from Beethoven's Symphony No. 9

"Jesu, Joy of Man's Desiring" by Johann Sebastian Bach

"Piano Sonata No. 16 in C Major

" (1st movement) by Wolfgang Amadeus Mozart

"Yellow Submarine" by The Beatles

"Sweet Home Alabama" by Lynyrd Skynyrd

"Can't Stop the Feeling!" by Justin Timberlake
"Viva la Vida" by Coldplay
"Hey, Soul Sister" by Train

There are hundreds of scales around the world created and established.

In a nutshell, every scale is a one-of-a-kind masterpiece, offering its own distinct flavor and vibe. Exploring the various scales is an adventure, especially when delving into non-Western musical scales and crafting unique, unconventional sets.

Understanding the characteristics of different scales and keys can be a game changer when crafting a specific atmosphere in a sound bath or when facilitating vibrational therapy for people.

Top composers meticulously select their scales and keys to elicit the desired emotions and to convey their artistic message to the audience. The possibilities are endless, and the journey of discovery is endlessly fascinating, especially when mixed into the realm of healing and therapeutics.

For beginners, it's best to start by getting familiar with the major diatonic scale and its format. Once you've got that down, move on to the minor scale and then to the pentatonic, and feel free to experiment from there.

Nowadays, I find myself on the internet for answers

to questions like, "What music scale was a favorite by certain composers ?" or "What's the most popular musical scale in India?" What are some forgotten scales, are there records of scales in biblical text, hidden archive scales, banned scales and so on.

KEYS

A musical key is a way to describe the overall sound, feeling, or mood of a piece of music. It revolves around a specific tonal center and a tonic note, usually called a "home note." The concept of key helps musicians understand which notes and chords sound well together in a particular song, and it also helps with composing and improvising. Each key is named after the main note, also called the root note and tonic. For example, the key of C major is based on the note C, C being the tonic.. For example, the key of C major uses the natural notes C, D, E, F, G, A, and B. Playing these notes in sequence creates a specific mood, with C being the home note. By playing the C major scale's first, third, and fifth notes, you get the C major chord, CEG, which is also part of the C primary key.

Think of times that a song or an instrument made you feel something. Maybe it made you feel happy, sad, or melancholic. This is usually because of the key the composer chose; in that key, there are specific notes, intervals, scales, and chords. To better understand what a key is in music, let's compare the twelve notes of the chromatic scale, which is what Crystal Tones® uses and labels on their bowls, to items in our fridge.

Imagine you have twelve different ingredients in your fridge. You could randomly throw them all together, and it might taste good or not. There's a lot of room for error in that approach. Now, imagine you have a specific recipe in mind, so you know that it requires certain ingredients, and you pull out the elements you need to make your dish. Let's say you're making a cake with a particular flavor; let's go with chocolate. The seven ingredients you will use as the basis of the recipe (eggs, flour, sugar, etc.) are like the notes within a key that form specific scales and chords. So, the final result, the cake, in that case, is the musical key, a sum that tastefully combines everything. If you add chocolate, it gives the cake a particular flavor. There are other flavors, like banana, carrot, or blueberries, and these are the key ingredients that provide a unique flavor to your cake.

In this analogy, the twelve ingredients in the fridge represent the twelve notes in the chromatic scale. Choosing a specific set of seven ingredients for your recipe requires the notes to create a particular scale and chords in music. The final result of the recipe, the cake, represents the key, and the key ingredient, the chocolate, represents the overall flavor and mood of the key. The frequencies of each key resonate with the human ear differently, making us feel that there is a different mood and taste in every key. Some Alchemy bowls™ will naturally complement each other based on their notes and frequencies, while others may clash or create dissonance.

TRIADS AND CHORDS

A music chord is a group of three or more notes in a chosen scale played together. Groups of three notes played at the same time are called **triads**. Groups of 3 or more notes played simultaneously are called **chords**. Both of these are the harmonic foundation of a key and are essential in harmonizing melodies.

A chord can be played on a single polyphonic instrument or by multiple instruments or voices.

Let's use a practical example to understand this analogy. We will take the C major scale and form the **tonic chord**, which is the C major chord. The notes of the C major scale are:

C D E F G A B C

To form the C major triad, take the **scale's first, third, and fifth** notes. You will end up with C, E, and G. Play all these simultaneously and have a C major chord.

CHORD PROGRESSIONS

Every key consists of a combination of major, minor, and diminished chords that work well together and sound good if played one after the other. The order in which chords are played is called **chord progression**.

When building a singing bowl set, knowing the difference between chord types can be helpful. If the first bowl you pick for your set is a note D, you should research the musical characteristics of the key of D major and D minor or any that start with d . This doesn't have to be a deciding factor, but it can help you learn how and why using the key of D has inspired others to feel for centuries.

Visualize your most beloved song. It likely adheres to a specific structure and format, and it has a particular chord progression complemented by a repeating chorus and a definitive emotional impact. The chosen key and rhythm serve as the backbone structure of the song; the chord progression sets the harmonic foundation of the song, while the scale chosen dictates what notes the melodies will sound like in the song. Everything, put together, provides the mood and essence of the song.

Applying this knowledge to singing bowl sets is helpful. For instance, a seven-bowl set could be built based on the major or minor scale. The pentatonic scale would be an ideal choice if a more straightforward five-bowl set is desired. If a three-bowl set is preferred, utilizing the primary chord of the chosen scale would be perfect.

Let me tell you how this relates to the decision process with Alchemy Bowls™. Imagine your friend or client, etc., has asked you to build a three-bowl set that is musically cohesive and emotionally evocative of darker, somber tones that can take someone on a journey through grief. You could research music scales and keys known to produce such emotions to accomplish this.

After a bit of research, you will come across two scales that may be suitable for your client's needs:

1. **D Flat Major**
2. **D Major**

Since the request was for a three-bowl set, you will likely build a chord from one of these scales. So, you need to identify the root chord associated with each.

The root chord of D Flat Major is made from the notes Db, F, and Ab, while the chord for D Major is D, F#, and A.

We went over how to form triads and chord progressions, but if you need help with this, you can easily find this information online by searching for the chords each key consists of.

Now that you have two options for your friend's or client's three-bowl set, you must consider building that first set with flats.

But how would you build a D-flat chord when the labels on the Alchemy bowls™ don't include flats?

The first note we need for the Db flat major chord is Db. It is a half step *lower* than the note D and played on a black key which is C#.

The second note we need is an F, which is simple enough, and the third is an Ab. Ab is one-half step *lower* than the note A, played on a black key. We have the note G# So, the bowls you need to build a three-set bowl of the Db major chord are C#, F, and G#.

Feel free to use the chakra or piano pictures to understand this more easily. It's essential to consider the sound's direction, whether it ascends or descends, and any desired transitions.

For example, to achieve an ascending order, you can make the C# bowl a 9-inch, the F bowl an 8-inch, and the G# bowl a 7-inch. This arrangement gradually increases the pitch and allows the bowls to stack seamlessly together, as usually, three bowls can fit into one case.

While knowledge and understanding of basic music theory concepts are important they shouldn't limit your creativity, imagination, or intentions behind your or your client's desires.

The Circle of Fifths is a diagram showing the relationships between major and minor keys in Western music and the key signature of each key (how many sharps or flats it has).

THE CIRCLE OF FIFTHS

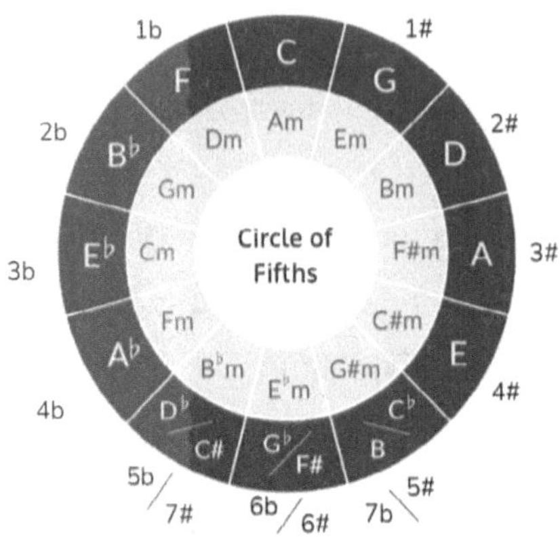

The outer circle in black has all the primary keys, while the inner circle in gray has all the minor keys. If you read the Circle of Fifths clockwise, you will see that the sharps are adding up until 7, and if you read it counter-clockwise, the flats are adding up until 7. This means that the G primary key has one sharp, the D major key has two sharps, and so on. Conversely, the F major key has one flat, the Bb major key has two flats, and so on.

To quickly find which notes are sharpened or flattened in a key, you need to follow the order of the sharps for keys on the right side of the Circle of Fifths or the order of flats for keys on the left side.

If learning here about the circle of fifths still confuses you, I suggest watching a YouTube or other online explanation. If you don't care to learn it but still want to dive right into the scales and chords and have them handed to you, refer to the set building chapter.

TUNING STANDARDS

The goal of tuning is to achieve a uniform pitch standard that can be used on different instruments and across various genres of music. In the Western world, the most commonly used tuning system is A440 tuning. This is widely referred to as equal temperament tuning. To achieve A440 tuning, the A note is tuned to a frequency of 440 Hz. Alchemy bowls™ have a number next to the note, such as A+40 or A-15. This number represents cents and refers to the deviation from the standard tuning frequency of True tone (440 Hz). Which would be AO

The establishment of A440 as a pitch standard is credited to an international conference in London in 1939, where delegates from various countries agreed on this standard. However, it took several decades for A440 to become widely accepted as the tuning standard in classical music performances and recordings. Today, A440 is the most commonly used tuning standard in Western music, and it is used as a reference point for tuning musical instruments. Instruments such as the piano, guitar, violin, viola, cello, double bass, flute, clarinet, and timpani are typically tuned to A440 Hz. Interestingly enough, brass

Instruments like the trumpet, saxophone, trombone, and tuba are tuned at 442Hz instead of 440Hz.

Different musical traditions and genres use other tuning systems. If you want to play alongside other instruments, ensure your instruments are tuned based on the same tuning standard.

There are many different opinions on why the A440 tuning system became established, but I'm not going to get into those here as it can get into the conspiracy realm.

On the majority of singing bowls, you will find that each bowl is labeled with a letter (the note name), a number, and a plus or minus sign. Let's see how that works. A perfect pitch true tone bowl would be labeled with a zero next to the letter. For example A0, B0, D0. If the number next to the letter has a plus sign (A+15), the note is slightly sharper, closer to the next note on the chromatic scale. For example, if the A note is in the +40 cents range, it is closer to A#.

On the other hand, if the number has the minus sign (A-15), the note is slightly flatter, closer to the following note down on the chromatic scale. The majority of practitioners consider any bowl where the cent range is within 10 from zero, either positive or negative, as a true tone.. So, the number zero next to the note, which we'll refer to as true tone, means that the note is ideally in tune with the established A440 tuning system.

When building sets according to music theory, it's not mandatory but it's good to ensure that all the Bowls are as close as possible to the exact cent. If you have a set of notes, such as A, C, and E. You would want all the notes to be within the same cent range, whether 0, + 5, -20, etc. Theoretically, the closer they are all to the same number, the more in harmony they sound.

Playing with musical pitch can significantly impact the overall sound and feel of a piece. When different notes are not in harmony, the result can be jarring and dissonant, taking away from the pleasantly intended musical experience. This is why the idea of mixing positive and negative cents can be met with skepticism by some.

However, this is not to say that experimentation and exploration should be discouraged. As creative beings, we should not limit ourselves to preconceived notions or established sets of information. In fact, some of the most exciting and innovative musical works have come from pushing boundaries and venturing into new territory. So, while mixing positive and negative cents may lead to dissonance, it can also lead to unexpected and exciting results that enhance the music's overall sound and emotional impact. The key is approaching these experiments with an open mind, a willingness to take risks, and a commitment to the creative process.

I recommend taking a break before we continue.

In the past, I was confused when individuals requested a complete set of bowls in varying shapes and sizes, all calibrated to either 528 hertz, 440, or 432 hertz. I was conflicted for 2 reasons. One is that for a bowl to be exactly 432 hertz it would have to be a specific size and note that = 432hz so if they wanted a whole set that way wouldn't that make it so everybowl had to be the same ? I was also conflicted because I was taught that all the bowls in the negative range of minus 20 to 40 were 432 Hz, while those in the positive cent range of 20 to 50 were 528 Hz and didn't matter the size, shape etc .

When I checked the tuning app on my phone, a bowl marked C-20, for example wasn't 432 hertz even though its within that range of -20-40. Instead it showed a specific frequency depending on the bowl's size, shape, and note somewhere within the range of 200-600. This left me questioning how I could build a set of bowls of different shapes and sizes yet have them all calibrated to 432.

I was overthinking it, and I was confused.

I eventually learned that tuning systems as a whole are different from specific hertz values. It's important to note that when instruments, like pianos, guitars, and singing bowls are tuned around A440, it doesn't mean all the bowls, keys or strings are A440 Hz. The A440 serves as a reference point within that particular tuning system. The fact that most singing bowls are tuned in reference to

A440 that's why any bowl that has a 0 next to the note is considered true tone and aligns in reference within that tuning system.

When you encounter a bowl with a negative cent value from -20 to -40, it corresponds closer to the 432-hertz tuning system because you are going negative from the traditional A440. Conversely, when you come across a bowl with a positive value from +20 to +50, it aligns more closely with 528-hertz tuning. The conversation revolves more around the tuning system and deviations of those tuning systems rather than the specific frequencies of each bowl themselves.

When aiming to create a whole set of bowls in the 432 tuning range, the approach would be to build the entire set with a cent range from -20 to -40. This means each bowl would be tuned slightly lower than the standard tuning of A440 as 432 is negative of 440. For a complete set of true-tone bowls, the goal would be to have all the bowls tuned at 0 or very close to it. This procedure ensures the bowls are tuned precisely according to the intended standard.

On the other hand, if the objective is to create a whole set in the 528 range, the approach would be to have all the bowls tuned in the +20 to +50 cent range. This means each bowl would be slightly pitch higher than the standard A440 tuning. True tone is considered equal temperament, and 432 is regarded as precise temperament tuning. 528 is not an official tuning system, but it is favored due to YouTube's popularity and also being a part of the Ancient solfeggio frequencies. The -20 to -40, + 20 to plus 50 is also a loose range. If you want each bowl to be extremely specific down to the very hertz that aligns with 440 or 432 tuning you can find these charts easily online.

BUILDING THE IDEAL SET FOR YOU

There are a lot of music theory concepts that you may take into consideration when building a set. These guidelines are meant to give answers to some of the most frequent music theory-related questions that one encounters when making a bowl set.

All the music theory concepts mentioned in this part of the book have been serving as the foundation of music for centuries, helping composers, songwriters, musicians, and performers reach their unique pinnacle in music. As mentioned at the beginning of this part, the basis of all music and music theory is frequencies, dynamics, and rhythm.

A tool that can always be useful in sound healing work is the concept of consonance and dissonance. Consonance refers to sounds that are harmonious and pleasing to the ear, while dissonance refers to harsh or unpleasant sounds. Both have their place in music. You can use dissonance or consonance to bring up someone held onto traumas or help calm someone's emotions when things do surface.

OCTAVES

Each singing usually has a sticker indicating its properties and a letter representing its musical note but not its octave. So, you might see two bowls with the same letter, but one bowl is big and one is small. What's the difference?

Both bowls are labeled with an A, but one sounds higher or lower than the other. In music this is referred to as an **octave**. If you divide the Frequency of that note in half, you get an octave lower. For example: A4, which is a 4th octave A, is at 440 Hz, and A3 (an octave lower) is at 220 Hz.

The term octave comes from the Latin word "octavus," meaning eighth. Pythagoras wasnt the first to try 8 notes but was the first to accomplish it without a huge conflict, for years 7 notes was established and to try anything other was pretty much heresy. On the far left of a piano, the keys have a lower sound, and as you move across the piano to the right, the notes get higher. A standard 88-key piano has 7 octaves.

For instance, if we take the A note, a larger alchemy bowl might produce a deep and soulful sound in the third octave, while a smaller bowl might produce a more angelic and higher-pitch sound in the 4th or 5th octave.

A piano might have 7 octaves, but the Alchemy bowls™ usually only range from the 3rd to the 5th octave.

As you've read earlier, each note has a corresponding frequency, measured in hertz (Hz). For example, the first note A has a frequency of 27.5 Hz. To move up to the A note in the first octave, the hertz is simply doubled to 55 Hz. This pattern continues with A2 at 110 Hz, A3 at 220 Hz, A4 at 440 Hz, etc.

Theoretically, this process could continue infinitely, but for practical purposes, most singing bowls fall within the 200 to 600 Hz range. People will consider the bowls between that range to sound low, mid, or high. Most crystal bowls range from 5 to 32 Inches, with the majority being 6-12 inches.

If someone asks me to find them a 3rd octave A bowl, I know I am going to be looking for a bigger, lower-tone bowl versus if they wanted a 5th octave A. I would need one of our smaller, high-pitch bowls.

To sum this up, the human voice typically has a range of about two octaves, although some singers can sing in three or more octaves. The range of audible frequencies for the human ears is between 20 Hz and 20,000 Hz, which spans over 10 octaves.

Humans can hear about 10 octaves, whereas a standard piano has 7 octaves. The range of most singing bowls falls within the 3rd to 5th octave. Somebigger crystal and metal bowls are in the second.   Then delete this tex after. and there might be lots of changes depending on what the future for the company holds and what they want to create.

IDEOLOGY

Sometimes, when we learn a set of information, we can become so attached to it that we trap ourselves within that knowledge, whether limited or vast. With singing bowls, this can sometimes be to our detriment. Let me give you an example: Someone wants a singing bowl for the throat chakra; the widely agreed-upon note for that is G.

You find a G bowl and play it for them, but they don't feel it in their throat – they feel it in their stomach. It's not beneficial to argue with or convince them they are wrong about where they should feel it. Sound bowls have dozens of layers to them, sound and vibration still extends far beyond the general understanding provided to the public.

Depending on various factors such as each person's emotional, physical, and spiritual density, where they might have blockages and trauma, their age, senses, and even down to the cells of their body, they experience life differently, as we all do. The system we have gone over are commonplace and widely accepted, but different parts of the world may use different music scales and relate them to the chakra system differently. They may say that G is not for the throat but for the solar plexus, and that's okay, too. The sounds and vibrations of the bowls will affect each of us personally, which should be celebrated and encouraged.

Perhaps the person you are helping listens to a C bowl for the root chakra, but they happen to feel it in their throat. This is a reminder to be open and adaptable, not rigid. Maybe they do feel it in their throat, what they have actually been afraid to speak about and vocalize is issues with stability in their relationship, which could be a root chakra issue.

There are a lot of possibilities and variations that go into it. You might build a set of bowls for someone, and after all the math, education, and tuning apps, you know that the set you made according to music theory is perfect, but the person doesn't like it or resonate with it. They might switch out one of the bowls for something completely off-tone and shouldn't work together, but to them, it's beautiful. This is perfectly fine since we all experience things in different ways.

CREDITS

From ancient civilizations like the Babylonians, Greeks, and Egyptians to the medieval and Renaissance periods in Western music, musicians and scholars have developed this complex system for centuries. These early civilizations used symbols to represent different musical pitches and rhythms, which evolved into today's music notation. In the Western world, music theory became more defined during the Medieval, Renaissance, and Baroque periods, where composers like Bach and Mozart began to create works that later defined the European musical tradition and influenced composers of the Romantic era, such as Beethoven.

One of the most significant figures in the development of this tuning system was

Andreas Werckmeister, a German organist and music theorist who lived in the late 17th century. He is known for creating a tuning system that allowed for more flexibility and compatibility between different keys, which became an essential foundation for the equal temperament system used in Western music today. To shed light on a few others:

Pythagoras is known for developing the Pythagorean tuning system, a method of tuning musical instruments based on the ratios of the lengths of strings. According to this system, the proportions of the lengths of strings that produce harmonious sounds are whole numbers. This system was significant because it introduced the concept of mathematical ratios to music and profoundly influenced the development of Western music theory.

Johann Sebastian Bach is famous for his keyboard works and compositions that utilized the tuning system known as "well-temperament."

Jean-Philippe Rameau was a French composer and music theorist in the 18th century and is known for his contributions to understanding harmony and tonality.

Heinrich Schenker was an Austrian music theorist in the early 20th century who developed a highly influential approach to analyzing tonal music known as "Schenkerian analysis."

Arnold Schoenberg, an Austrian composer in the early 20th century, is known for his development of atonal and development of serialist compositional techniques that challenged traditional tonal structures. These are just a few of the most notable examples, but many other prominent figures have contributed to the development of Western music.

Chapter 7

CRATING SETS

WHAT ARE SETS

A set typically consists of two or more singing bowls intentionally selected and played together to create a specific soundscape. Sets can be used for various purposes, including meditation, relaxation, Concerts, and different sound healing modalities. The typical sets are 3 bowl sets, 3 and a 4th bowl added sometimes to complete the octave, 5 bowl sets, 7 bowl sets, and 12 bowl Symphony sets.

WHY IS BUILDING SETS IMPORTANT

First, it allows practitioners to create specific soundscapes for their clients. By intentionally selecting bowls with complementary tones and frequencies, practitioners can create a blend of sounds that can induce a meditative or activating state for different types of work based on the intention.

Secondly, building sets can help practitioners tailor their practice to meet the specific needs of their clients.

Different clients may require different approaches to sound healing therapy, and building custom sets can help practitioners create personalized sessions that target their clients' unique needs. Moreover, building sets allow practitioners to explore the unique properties of different bowls and experiment with different combinations of tones, frequencies, Alchemies, chakras, etc. This can lead to new insights and discoveries about the therapeutic potential of sound and can help practitioners continuously improve their practice.

TYPES OF SETS

<u>Harmonics.</u>

Harmonics refers to the combination of multiple frequencies that occur simultaneously and create a musical or sound-like pattern. We all know how music can affect us in different ways. Some songs can make us cry, others can make us angry or upset, and some can make us feel calm and relaxed. Frequencies of music and other external sounds can have a direct impact on our physical and emotional well-being. Each of our cells vibrates at its own frequency, so it's no surprise that the Frequency of external sounds can influence us in many ways.

<u>Chakras.</u>

One way to Build sets and utilize singing bowls is by aligning them with specific chakras. For instance, Most singing bowls are designated to the various chakras shown below.

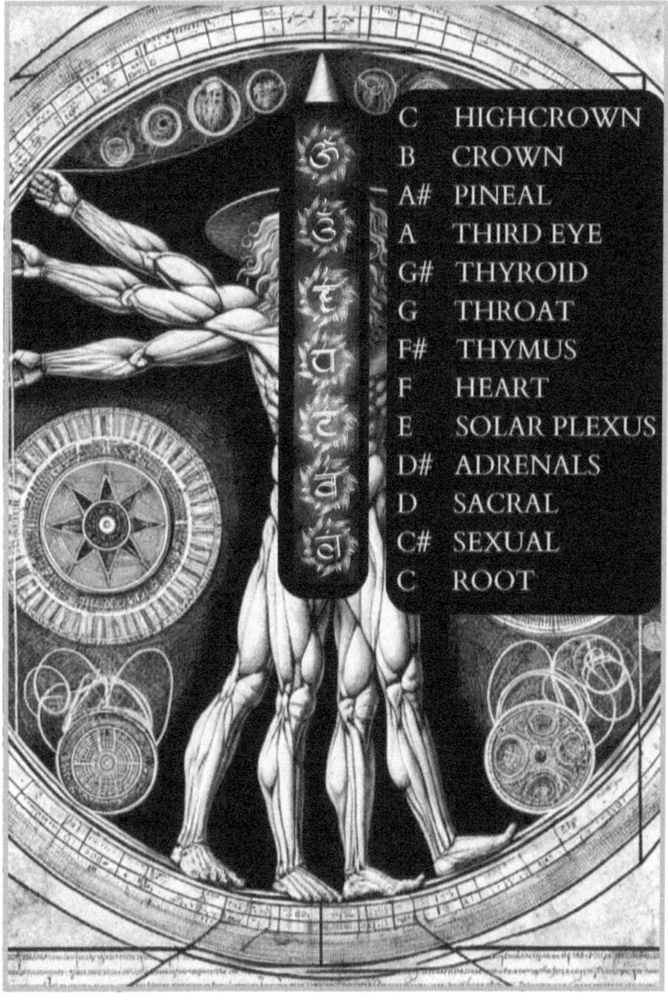

When building a set of singing bowls with specific chakras in mind most people prioritize C,D,E,F,G,A,B for each main chakra or a endocrine set C#,D#,F#,G#,A#. They would select these from low to high meaning bigger bowls to smaller bowls. If they only wanted 3 bowls they might go for the root, heart and third eye or sacral, throat and crown.

I would add and emphasize here that it's more important to go from low to high in a chakra set to get energy moving and flowing than rigidly starting with a particular note. A chakra set doesn't have to start with C. A chakra set could start with A or any of the notes as long as you go from low to high meaning low hertz to high hertz, grounding to angelic, relaxing to stimulating etc. Some people who focus specifically on the chakra system are usually more focused on the chakras and might care less about specific properties, music theory, and other modalities when building their sets.

Alchemies

Some people build sets Solely around the alchemies as Alchemy takes center stage at Crystal Tones®, where decades of energy, time, and dedication have converged to birth the signature Alchemy bowls™, each an embodiment of pure intention.

Crystals

Some people may deeply connect to certain crystals and want to incorporate them into their sound healing practice. For example, amethyst is known for its calming and soothing properties, while citrine is associated with abundance and manifestation. Rose quartz is often used for heart healing, and black tourmaline is believed to help protect against negative energy. Each of these crystals has more in-depth and specific uses.

When selecting singing bowls created with specific crystals, one approach is to choose bowls that have similar properties to the crystals. For instance, you might pair an amethyst bowl tuned to the note A, which is associated with the third eye chakra and is believed to help with intuition and spiritual growth.

Another approach is to select singing bowls that complement the crystal's energy. For for example, you might pair rose quartz with an alchemy bowl that is tuned to the note F, which is associated with the heart chakra and is believed to promote feelings of love and compassion.

Intuition

This method for creating a set is to rely on intuition and personal preferences when selecting the bowls.

This approach prioritizes channeling and intuition over the technical aspects of sound harmonization.

This process involves allowing oneself or the client to explore various singing bowls until a set of bowls that resonates with their personal energy and preferences is identified.

These preferences may include factors such as the bowls' size, shape, weight, material, and sound. By relying on intuition, the practitioner can select a set of bowls that align with the client's energy and resonate with their needs and preferences.

While this method does not guarantee a technically harmonious sound, the focus is on creating a set of bowls that channels the right energy. As such, this approach is popular among energy healers, spiritual practitioners, and individuals seeking a personalized and intuitive approach to sound healing. The owner of Crystal Tones Lupito Built sets for clients like this successfully for over 2 decades.

Binaural

It's made by playing two slightly different bowls at the same time. For example, they will create a binaural beat if you play a 9" A+30 bowl and a 9" A-30 bowl together. This auditory illusion is created by the brain when it tries to process both tones at the same time. Some people believe that binaural beats can help healing because our brains tend to sync up with external stimuli, like sound waves.

Proponents of binaural beat therapy believe that when the brain is exposed to specific frequencies, it can become synchronized and balanced, Balancing the left and right hemispheres of the brain, leading to improved physical and emotional health while also being used to access different brain states dependent on the binaural. To create a set using binaural beats, it is recommended to select bowls of the same size and note but with slightly different cent values. This difference in cents is what helps to create the desired binaural beat effect.

This will sound like a wobble.

1. Beta Waves (12-30 Hz): This is the normal waking state of the brain when we are alert and attentive, and actively engaged in mental activity such as problem-solving, decision-making, and concentration.

2. Alpha Waves (8-12 Hz): This is a relaxed state of the brain, often associated with a meditative or reflective state, daydreaming, or light relaxation. It is commonly seen when the eyes are closed, but the person is not sleeping.

    1. Theta Waves (4-8 Hz): This is a deeper state of relaxation, often associated with a meditative or creative state, commonly seen during light sleep, meditation, or hypnosis.

    1. Delta Waves (0.5-4 Hz): This is the slowest brain wave frequency and is typically seen during deep sleep when the body is repairing and rejuvenating itself.

1. Gamma Waves (30-100 Hz): This is a high-frequency brain wave state that is associated with high-level cognitive processing, such as problem-solving, perception, and consciousness.

Brain states can shift rapidly and dynamically depending on the individual's current activity, environment, and internal state.

To determine which brain state you are trying to activate with the binaural beat you have created, you can use a tuner app to measure the Frequency of the two bowls. For example, if the first bowl plays at 220Hz (9" A0), and the second bowl plays at 225Hz (9" A-30), the difference between the two frequencies is 5Hz. According to the Frequency ranges mentioned earlier, this would fall under the theta brain state, associated with frequencies between 4 and 8 Hz.

True Tone

We addressed this in the music theory chapter.

The True Tone system was designed to help musicians tune their instruments to play alongside each other. It used unique technology that measured the exact frequency of each note and made precise adjustments to ensure every sound was in tune.

432hz

432 Hertz tuning is believed by some to offer numerous benefits over the standard 440 Hertz (true tone) Frequency commonly used in Western music. Proponents of 432 Hz tuning argue that it has a more natural and harmonious sound better suited to the human ear.

One of the main reasons why 432 Hz is considered beneficial is its relationship to nature. Many natural phenomena, such as the planets' movement and the earth's vibrations, are said to resonate at or near 432 Hz.

This has led some to suggest that 432 Hz is the true "natural" tuning Frequency and has a profound and positive effect on the human body and mind.

Some cool details about the benefits of 432 Hz include:

Research has shown that listening to music tuned to 432 Hz can lower heart rate and blood pressure, promote relaxation, and reduce anxiety and stress.

Many famous composers, including Mozart and Verdi, are said to have tuned their music to 432 Hz.

Some studies suggest that 432 Hz tuning can positively affect plant growth and help promote healing in the body. Many ancient cultures, such as the Egyptians and Greeks are believed to have used 432 Hz tuning in their music and instruments.

Overall, while the benefits of 432 Hz tuning are still debated in the music community, many people find the idea of a more natural and harmonious tuning frequency appealing and intriguing.

To build sets in 432 hertz Tuning, it would be any Crystal Tones® Alchemy Bowl in the negative cent range (-). Usually from -20 to - 40 on the bowls.

528HZ

The 528 Hertz tuning frequency, also known as the "Love Frequency," is believed by some to have numerous healing properties and benefits. Proponents of 528 Hz tuning argue that it can help to repair DNA, promote emotional balance and well-being, and facilitate spiritual growth. Some cool details about the benefits of 528 Hz include:

Research has shown that listening to music tuned to 528 Hz can increase the production of the neurotransmitter serotonin, which is associated with feelings of happiness and well-being. 528 Hz resonates at the heart chakra, associated with love, compassion, and emotional healing. Some studies suggest that 528 Hz tuning can repair DNA and restore it to its natural, healthy state. Many proponents of 528 Hz tuning believe it has a powerful and positive effect on the body's energy centers, or chakras.

Overall, while the benefits of 528 Hz tuning are still debated in the scientific and music communities, many people find the idea of a frequency that promotes love, healing, and emotional balance to be profoundly appealing and powerful.

Solfeggio Frequencies

The origins of the Solfeggio frequencies can supposedly be traced back to the medieval hymn "Ut queant laxis," where each line of the hymn begins with a successive note of the musical scale. These would be certain vowel sounds you could chant that match specific frequencies which help to naturally reset and heal parts of yourself that are out of alignment. Certain mystery schools go pretty in depth with these teachings, there is also quite a bit of information about how to do them on youtube and the internet. I might go more in depth here in my next body of work but for the sake of this we will keep it simple.

Guido of Arezzo, a Benedictine monk, is credited with the development of the solmization system, which eventually evolved into the familiar do-re-mi syllables we recognize today. The Solfeggio frequencies, as we know them, were rediscovered in the 20th century by Dr. Joseph Puleo and Dr. Leonard Horowitz. They stumbled upon a series of six frequencies that, when aligned with the traditional scale, created a harmonic believed to possess unique healing properties. I've also seen them go up to 9.

174 Hz - This frequency is associated with the natural order of life and is believed to be a powerful tool for grounding and establishing a sense of security and stability

285 Hz -Thought to enhance cognitive functions and facilitate the expansion of consciousness, 285 Hz is considered a bridge to higher states of awareness.

396 Hz -This frequency is often linked to the release of fear, guilt, and shame. It is believed to liberate the listener from negative emotions.

417 Hz - Associated with undoing situations and facilitating change,

417 Hz is thought to help break destructive patterns and promote positive transformation.

528 Hz - Widely recognized as the "Love Frequency," 528 Hz is believed to promote healing, repair DNA, and restore equilibrium in both the physical and spiritual realms.

639 Hz - This frequency is associated with the enhancement of interpersonal relationships, promoting communication, understanding, and unity.

741 Hz - Thought to detoxify the body and mind, 741 Hz is often linked to the purification of cells and the removal of toxins.

852 Hz Associated with intuition and spiritual insight, 852 Hz is believed to open the third eye and enhance one's

connection with the higher realms.

As you can see this is pretty much the same information as chakra work except this is more of the math behind it. You can use vowel sounds to hit each of these frequencies and is how people would heal themselves. You can also build sets in this hertz range although you would need to make some minor adjustments as most bowls dont go past 600 hertz. A way to do this would be to build with 174, 285, 396, 417, 528, then for 639, 741, 852 you could either use tuning forks which hold those frequencies or you could, half the frequencies and still build it with bowls. Half of 639 is 319.5, half of 741 is 370.5, half of 852 is 426 which you could all find with Alchemy bowls™ and your tuning app. The reason this works is because it's the same number, just a lower octave but still captures the essence.

One of the first things I found interesting with these numbers is that they are all the same numbers. 174,417,741 etc. When you input this in any kind of system where numbers generate patterns it creates Shapes such as the flower of life. So by using these that's what you are entraining yourself too.

<u>BEADGCF</u>

Everything we have discussed so far has mostly been in line with what companies such as Crystal tones® and other sound healing companies, courses, teachers etc have established. The tuning system in relation to the piano and chakras as well as what was taught by the vedic system. "Vedic" refers to anything related to the Vedas, which are a collection of ancient sacred texts that form the foundation of Hindu religious and philosophical traditions. The Vedas are among the oldest religious scriptures in the world and are considered the most authoritative and revered texts in Hinduism.

But there is another system some call it the Tibetan system BEADGCF (that's from high to low)with b being the crown e being the third eye a being the throat d,heart g, solar plexus c, sacral and f being the root. People have come up with lots of abbreviations for what this means but the most traditional is BEAD G(god) C (Comes) F(First).

The Vedic tradition is predominantly associated with Hinduism and its scriptures, while the Tibetan tradition is primarily linked to Tibetan Buddhism and the broader Buddhist tradition.

Guitar players also use this pattern, here is a interesting link that further goes into depth Lesson 8: The BEAD-GCF Pattern | Guitar Theory Revolution.

One reason I personally like occasionally using this system is because of all the research, studies and benefits of intervals of 5ths in music. How it is especially pleasing and helps one into a state of relaxation. This system is a full chakra system built off of intervals of 5ths. You would start with the root. F being the biggest bowl and working up, 5 notes up is C 5 up from there is G etc.

Benefits of Perfect Fifths

Perfect fifths contribute to harmonic stability and are considered consonant intervals; they are also needed for building chords. In triads, the combination of a root, third, and fifth forms the basic major or minor chord, influencing the overall sound and quality of the chord. The concept of the circle of fifths is also fundamental in music theory. It illustrates the relationship between key signatures, chord progressions, and modulation, providing a tool for understanding tonal relationships.

The perfect fifth is associated with specific chakras. Each chakra is believed to correspond to a specific musical note, and the perfect fifth is often linked to the heart chakra (Anahata). Using this interval is thought to support the alignment and balance of the heart chakra. So by building a set this way you could focus each chakra with every note also working on the heart, Relaxation and Stress Reduction. The perfect fifth is present in various natural sounds, such as the calls of certain birds or the sounds of wind and water. Aligning with these natural frequencies is believed to have a grounding and calming effect.

Pythagoras' Contribution:

- Mathematical Ratios:
- Pythagoras, an ancient Greek philosopher and mathematician, explored the mathematical ratios of musical intervals. He is credited with the Pythagorean tuning system, where intervals are derived from simple ratios of whole numbers, such as the 3:2 ratio for the perfect fifth.
- Foundational Work:
- Pythagoras laid the foundation for understanding the mathematical relationships governing musical intervals. His work on ratios and proportions influenced the development of music theory and tuning systems in ancient Greece, shaping the way intervals like the perfect fifth were conceptualized and applied in Western musical traditions.

SET BUILDING STRATEGIES

As a Certified sound healer and an experienced practitioner, The objective is to consistently maintain the highest standard when building and assembling sets, thus setting a quality benchmark in the industry.

While some customers may prioritize specific chakras or crystals and may not be as concerned about harmonious combinations or tuning, we ensure that every set built has the highest level of intention and can match as many layers as possible.

GUIDELINES TO FOLLOW WHILE BUILDING

To create a set that aligns with a vision for yourself or a client:

1. **Listening to their story, asking questions, and understanding their vision.**

2. **Cent range: Keeping all the bowls you pick within 20 cents of each other Unless intentional or creating a binaural. This is a rule of thumb, but don't sandbox yourself; every bowl is unique, and I've found bowls that play beautifully together outside the set range. Make sure not to make this another rigid belief system. Play, have fun, experiment.**

3. **Find a chord or music scale that complements their requests. This doesn't necessarily mean that you should offer them a package of music scales, but rather that you should personally consider which scales would work well together when building their set.**

4. **Aesthetic: creating an aesthetic that the client is happy with.**

5. **The cherry on top: If building a 3, 5, 7, or 12 bowl set, always present it with the next bowl in the chord or complete the octave. This is the finishing touch that adds that extra layer of love.**

6. **When building a set of bowls, remember that typically, 3 bowls fit in a case. Creating a set that**

ascends or descends the scale from low to high or high to low is generally preferred. The bowl considered the cherry on top is usually a small bowl, considered a high note. For example, if your set consists of a 9" C, 8" E, and 7" G, they would stack nicely, and then you could add the 6" C to complete the octave and add the finishing touch.

<u>Tools to Help You Build Sets</u>

Resources that can make set building easier, including apps, educational materials, and consulting services

N- Track Tuner is a free app that you can download. It will tell you the exact octave, cent range, hertz, and note the bowl is playing you can also change the default setting if you want to build cents in different tuning ranges

Here is a list of popular music scales and how they can be constructed using Singing Bowls. Many music scales contain flats, but most bowls dont show flats.

Therefore, I have provided conversions and instructions on how to build sets using Alchemy bowls™, even for those scales that include flats. Here are some ideas for 3 Bowl sets:

3 BOWL SETS

The addition of the 4th bowl is not necessary, but highly recommended to complete the octave and create more movement. This is especially true when ascending from a low to high.

C

C Major C - E - G - c. <u>Bright, happy, uplifting, Joy, calm</u>

C Minor C - D# - G - c. <u>Sad, melancholic, introspection, tension.</u>

C#

C# major C# - E# - G# -c#. <u>Bright, powerful, bold, confident.</u>

C# Minor C# - E - G# - c#. <u>Dark, brooding, intensity.</u>

D

D Major D - F# - A - d. <u>Optimism, celebration, upbeat, lively.</u>

D Minor D - F- A - d. <u>Nostalgia, reflection, somber.</u>

D#

D# Major D# - G - A# - d#. <u>Triumphant, excitement, strength.</u>

D# Minor D# - F# - A# - d#. <u>Dark journey, moody, melancholy.</u>

E

E Major E - G# - B - e. <u>Hopefulness, empowerment, victory.</u>

E minor E - G - B - e. <u>Longing, yearning, reflectiveness.</u>

F

F Major F- A - C - f. <u>Playfulness, warmth, elation, radiance.</u>

F Minor F - G# - C -f. <u>Sentimentality, tenderness, longing.</u>

F#

F# Major F - A - C - f#. <u>Heroism, vitality, thrill.</u>

F# Minor F# - A - C# - f#. <u>Vulnerability, anguish, tragedy.</u>

G

G Major G - B - D -g. <u>Fun, bliss, freedom.</u>

G Minor G - A# - D -g. <u>Grief, loneliness, mourning.</u>

G#

G# major G# - B# - D# - g#. <u>Confidence, expansive, majestic.</u>

G# minor G# - B - D# - g#. <u>Dramatic, contemplative, tragic.</u>

A

A major A - C - E - a. <u>Serenity, youthful, romantic.</u>

A minor A - C- E -a. <u>Pensive, mysterious contemplation.</u>

<u>A#</u>

A# major A# - C - F - a#. <u>Sunny, festive, inspiring.</u>

A# minor A# -C# - F - a#. <u>Poignant, wistful, pensive.</u>

<u>B</u>

B Major

B - D# - F# - b. <u>Simple, happy, fresh.</u>

B Minor

B - D - F# - b. <u>Desolation, sentimentality, lamentation.</u>

5 Bowl Sets Following the Pentatonic Scale.

MAJORS

- C major pentatonic scale: C-D-E-G-A (Happy, joyful, optimistic)
- C# major pentatonic scale: C#-D#-F-G#-A# (Mystical, dreamy, enchanted)
- D major pentatonic scale: D-E-F#-A-B (Joyful, triumphant, energetic)
- D# major pentatonic scale: D#-F-G-A#-C (Mysterious, exotic, alluring)
- E major pentatonic scale: E-F#-G#-B-C# (Uplifting, hopeful, inspiring)
- F major pentatonic scale: F-G-A-C-D (Serene, calming, peaceful)
- F# major pentatonic scale: F#-G#-A#-C#-D# (Exciting, adventurous, playful)
- G major pentatonic scale: G-A-B-D-E (Peaceful, calm, soothing)

- G# major pentatonic scale: G#-A#-C-D#-F (Mysterious, intriguing, seductive)
- A major pentatonic scale: A-B-C#-E-F# (Hopeful, uplifting, inspiring)
- A# major pentatonic scale: A#-C-D#-F-G# (Dark, dramatic, mysterious)
- B major pentatonic scale: B-C#-D#-F#-G# (Energetic, upbeat, enthusiastic)

MINORS

- A minor pentatonic scale: A-C-D-E-G (Mysterious, contemplative, haunting)
- A# minor pentatonic scale: A#-C#-D#-F#-G# (Moody, dark, mysterious)
- B minor pentatonic scale: B-D-E-F#-A (Reflective, melancholic, introspective)
- C minor pentatonic scale: C-D#-F-G-A# (Eerie, spooky, foreboding)
- C# minor pentatonic scale: C#-E-F#-G#-B (Intense, passionate, dramatic)
- D minor pentatonic scale: D-F-G-A-C (Melancholic, pensive, wistful)
- D# minor pentatonic scale: D#-F#-G#-A#-C# (Sultry, dark, emotional)
- E minor pentatonic scale: E-G-A-B-D (Mysterious, haunting, introspective)
- F minor pentatonic scale: F-G#-A#-C-D# (Brooding, introspective, melancholic)
- F# minor pentatonic scale: F#-A-B-C#-E (Passionate, intense, moody)

- G minor pentatonic scale: G-A#-C-D-F (Sad, melancholic, wistful)
- G# minor pentatonic scale: G#-B-C#-D#-F# (Intense, moody, emotional)

Cultural Pentatonic Scales

The Ritusen Pentatonic Scale (Japanese)

C-D-E-G-A (whole tone, whole tone, minor third, whole tone)

Emotions: Majestic, evocative, tranquil

Cultural Association: Traditional Japanese music, Japanese folk songs and classical music

The Mongolian Pentatonic Scale (Mongolian)

A-B-C-E-F# (whole tone, whole tone, minor third, whole tone)

Emotions: Wistful, contemplative, haunting

Cultural Association: Mongolian traditional music, throat singing

The Egyptian Pentatonic Scale (Egyptian)

D-D#-F-A-A# (minor third, whole tone, whole tone, minor third)

Emotions: Exotic, mysterious, foreboding

Cultural Association: Ancient Egyptian music, Middle Eastern music

The Pelog Pentatonic Scale (Indonesian)

C-D-E-G-A#

Emotions: Meditative, spiritual, reflective

Cultural Association: Javanese gamelan music, traditional Indonesian music

Zodiac Sign Pentatonic Scales

Aries: G Pentatonic Scale

. G-A-B-D-E

. Emotions: Energetic, assertive, passionate

Taurus: F# Pentatonic Scale

. F#-G#-A#-C#-D#

. Emotions: Sensual, grounding, luxurious

Gemini: Bb Pentatonic Scale

. A#-C-D-F-G

. Emotions: Playful, curious, versatile

Cancer: Ab Pentatonic Scale

. G#-A#-C#-D#-F#

. Emotions: Nurturing, sensitive, emotional

Leo: D Pentatonic Scale

. D-E-F#-A-B

. Emotions: Confident, dramatic, expressive

Virgo: Eb Pentatonic Scale

. D#-F-G-A#-C

. Emotions: Analytical, precise, structured

Libra: A Pentatonic Scale

. A-B-C#-E-F#

. Emotions: Harmonious, balanced, romantic

Scorpio: E Pentatonic Scale

. E-F#-G#-B-C#

. Emotions: Intense, passionate, transformative

Sagittarius: C Pentatonic Scale

. C-D-E-G-A

. Emotions: Adventurous, free-spirited, optimistic

Capricorn: B Pentatonic Scale

. B-C#-D#-F#-G#

. Emotions: Disciplined, ambitious, grounded

Aquarius: Db Pentatonic Scale

. C#-D#-F-G#-A#

. Emotions: Eccentric, unconventional, visionary

Pisces: Gb Pentatonic Scale

. F#-G#-A#-C#-D#

. Emotions: Dreamy, mystical, imaginative.

Deity Pentatonic Scales

Shiva Pentatonic Scale (Hinduism)

C-D-E-G-A

Emotions: Meditative, mystical, transcendent

Cultural Association: Indian classical music, devotional music

Apollo Pentatonic Scale (Greek Mythology)

. C-D-E-G-A

Emotions: Poetic, radiant, noble

Cultural Association: Ancient Greek music, hymns and odes

Ra Pentatonic Scale (Egyptian Mythology)

E-F#-G#-B-C#

Emotions: Powerful, radiant, majestic

Cultural Association: Egyptian music, hymns and prayers

Amaterasu Pentatonic Scale (Shintoism)

C-C#-F-F#-G#

. Emotions: Radiant, uplifting, serene

Cultural Association: Japanese traditional music, Shinto music and rituals

Yahweh Pentatonic Scale (Judaism)

D-E-F#-A-B

Emotions: Majestic, awe-inspiring, transcendent

Cultural Association: Jewish liturgical music, psalms and hymns

Quetzalcoatl Pentatonic Scale (Aztec Mythology)

D-E-G-A-B

Emotions: Vibrant, spiritual, powerful

Cultural Association: Aztec music, rituals and ceremonies.

Odin Pentatonic Scale (Norse Mythology)

D-E-G-A-C

Emotions: Mysterious, powerful, wise

Cultural Association: Nordic music, ancient Scandinavian melodies and chants

Kuan Yin Pentatonic Scale (Buddhism)

G-A-B-D-E

Emotions: Calming, compassionate, serene

Cultural Association: Chinese Buddhist music, chants and hymns

Saraswati Pentatonic Scale (Hinduism)

C-D-E-G-B

Emotions: Creative, inspiring, meditative

Cultural Association: Indian classical music, devotional music and mantras

Christos Pentatonic Scale (Christianity)

E-F#-G#-B-C#

Emotions: Uplifting, peaceful, reverent

Cultural Association: Christian hymns and spirituals, sacred music

Inanna Pentatonic Scale (Sumerian Mythology)

E-F#-A-B-C#

Emotions: Passionate, powerful, sensual

Cultural Association: Sumerian music and poetry, ancient Near Eastern melodies

Quan Yin Pentatonic Scale (Taoism)

D-E-G-A-B

Emotions: Compassionate, tranquil, healing

Cultural Association: Chinese Taoist music, meditation, and healing practices.

Pentatonic Scales for the Seasons

Spring bhupala
A-A#-D-E F-

Spring Durga
A-B-D-E-F#-

Summer
C-D-E-G-A-

Summer

C-D-F-G-A#-

Rain season Vibhasa

F-F#-A-A#-B-D-

Autumn Malkaus

G-A#-C-D#-F-

Autumn Sri

G-G#-C-D-F#-

Winter Gunkali

D-D#-G-A-A#-

Winter Hindol

D-F#-G#-B-C#-

7 BOWL SETS

<u>C</u>

C Major Scale

C-D-E-F-G-A-B

Emotions: Happy, joyful, bright

Cultural Association: Western classical music, pop music, folk music

C Harmonic Minor Scale

C-D-D#-F-G-G#-B

Emotions: Dark, dramatic, passionate

Cultural Association: Western classical music, flamenco, jazz

C Lydian Scale

C-D-E-F#-G-A-B

Emotions: Mystical, dreamy, otherworldly

Cultural Association: Jazz, film music, psychedelic rock

C Dorian Scale

C-D-D#-F-G-A-A#

Emotions: Melancholic, contemplative, soulful

Cultural Association: Jazz, blues, pop music

C Mixolydian Scale

C-D-E-F-G-A-A#

Emotions: Groovy, bluesy, confident

Cultural Association: Rock music, blues, funk

Ionian Mode - C-D-E-F-G-A-B - Happy, joyful Calm

C Minor- C-D-D#-F-G-G#-A# - Dark, intense, brooding

Harmonic Major - C, D, E, F, G, G#, B - Mysterious, exotic

Double Harmonic - C-C#-E-F-G-G#-B - Enigmatic, dramatic

Hungarian Minor - C-C#-E-F#-G-G#-B - Exotic, tense

Spanish Gypsy - C-D-D#-F#-G-G#-B - Flamenco-inspired, passionate

Ukrainian Dorian - C-D-D#-F#-G-A-A# - Bittersweet, emotional

Blues Scale - C-D#-F-F#-G-A# - Sad, melancholic

Whole Tone - C-D-E-F#-G#-A# - Dreamy, mysterious

Chromatic - C-C#-D#-E-F#-G#-A#-B - Tense, suspenseful

Enigmatic - C-C#-E-F#-G#-A#-B - Mysterious, dramatic

Neapolitan Minor - C-C#-D#-F#-G-A-B - Dark, tense

Blues Minor - C-D#-F-F#-G-A# - Moody, bluesy

Blues Scale C-D#-F-A#-G-A#-C Sad, Bluesy, Soulful

Locrian: C-C#-D#-F-F#-G#-A#. dark and mysterious sound

C

C# Major Scale

    C#-D#-E#-F#-G#-A#-B#

    Emotions: Majestic, triumphant, grand

    Cultural Association: Classical music, film music, patriotic music

C# Minor Scale

    C#-D#-E-F#-G#-A-B

    Emotions: Melancholic, dramatic, intense

    Cultural Association: Classical music, heavy metal, hard rock

C# Harmonic Minor Scale

C#-D#-E-F#-G#-A-B#

Emotions: Mysterious, exotic, dramatic

Cultural Association: Flamenco, Middle Eastern music, heavy metal

C# Phrygian Scale

C#-D-E-F#-G#-A-A#

Emotions: Dark, moody, mysterious

Cultural Association: Flamenco, heavy metal, jazz

C# Locrian Scale

C#-D-E-F#-G-A-A#

Emotions: Unsettling, tense, ominous

Cultural Association: Avant-garde music, experimental music, jazz

<u>D</u>

D Major Scale

D-E-F#-G-A-B-C#

Emotions: Majestic, triumphant, joyful

Cultural Association: Classical music, pop music, folk music

D Minor Scale

D-E-F-G-A-A#-C#

Emotions: Melancholic, sad, intense

Cultural Association: Classical music, rock music, blues

D Lydian Scale

D-E-F#-G#-A-B-C#

Emotions: Dreamy, ethereal, optimistic

Cultural Association: Jazz, pop music, film music

D Mixolydian Scale

D-E-F#-G-A-B-C

Emotions: Bluesy, groovy, uplifting

Cultural Association: Rock music, blues, funk

D Phrygian Dominant Scale

D-E-F#-G#-A-B-C

Emotions: Exotic, intense, suspenseful

Cultural Association: Flamenco, Middle Eastern music, jazz

D#

D# Major Scale

D#-F-G-G#-A#-C-D

Emotions: Bright, cheerful, triumphant

Cultural Association: Classical music, pop music, electronic dance music

D# Minor Scale

D#-F-F#-G#-A#-B-C#

Emotions: Sad, melancholic, dramatic

Cultural Association: Classical music, rock music, blues

D# Phrygian Scale

D#-E-F#-G#-A#-B-C#

Emotions: Dark, mysterious, tense

Cultural Association: Flamenco, heavy metal, jazz

D# Locrian Scale

D#-E-F#-G#-A-B-C#

Emotions: Dissonant, unsettling, ominous

Cultural Association: Avant-garde music, experimental music, jazz

D# Double Harmonic Scale

D#-E-F -G -A -B-C

Emotions: Exotic, intense, dramatic

Cultural Association: Middle Eastern music, jazz, world music

E

E Major Scale

E-F#-G#-A-B-C#-D#

Emotions: Bright, joyful, triumphant

Cultural Association: Classical music, pop music, rock music

E Minor Scale

E-F#-G-A-B-C-D

Emotions: Melancholic, sad, introspective

Cultural Association: Classical music, rock music, blues

E Dorian Scale

E-F#-G-A-B-C#-D

Emotions: Mellow, dreamy, contemplative

Cultural Association: Jazz, pop music, folk music

E Phrygian Scale

E-F-G-A-B-C-D

Emotions: Dark, mysterious, exotic

Cultural Association: Flamenco, heavy metal, jazz

E Mixolydian Scale

E-F#-G#-A-B-C#-D

Emotions: Bluesy, groovy, uplifting

Cultural Association: Rock music, blues, funk

<u>F</u>

F Major Scale

F-G-A-A#-C-D-E

Emotions: Bright, triumphant, joyful

Cultural Association: Classical music, pop music, jazz

F Minor Scale

F-G-G#-A#-C-C#-D#

Emotions: Sad, melancholic, introspective

Cultural Association: Classical music, rock music, blues

F Lydian Scale

F-G-A-B-C-D-E

Emotions: Dreamy, mystical, ethereal

Cultural Association: Jazz, pop music, progressive rock

F Mixolydian Scale

F-G-A-A#-C-D-D#

Emotions: Groovy, bluesy, uplifting

Cultural Association: Rock music, blues, funk

F Phrygian Dominant Scale

F-F#-A-A#-C-C#-D#

Emotions: Exotic, intense, dramatic

Cultural Association: Middle Eastern music, jazz, world music

F#

F# Major Scale

F#-G#-A#-B-C#-D#-E#

Emotions: Bright, uplifting, triumphant

Cultural Association: Classical music, pop music, rock music

F# Minor Scale

F#-G#-A-B-C#-D-E

Emotions: Melancholic, introspective, dramatic

Cultural Association: Classical music, rock music, metal music

F# Dorian Scale

F#-G#-A-B-C#-D#-E

Emotions: Mellow, dreamy, introspective

Cultural Association: Jazz, pop music, folk music

F# Lydian Scale

F#-G#-A#-B#-C#-D#-E#

Emotions: Dreamy, uplifting, mystical

Cultural Association: Jazz, pop music, progressive rock

F# Mixolydian Scale

F#-G#-A#-B-C#-D#-E

Emotions: Groovy, bluesy, uplifting

Cultural Association: Rock music, blues, funk

G

G Major Scale:

G, A, B, C, D, E, F#

Emotions: Bright, joyful, triumphant

Cultural Association: Classical music, pop music, rock music

G Minor Scale: G, A, A#, C, D, D#, F

Emotions: Sad, melancholic, introspective

Cultural Association: Classical music, rock music, metal music

G Dorian Scale: G, A, A#, C, D, E, F

Emotions: Mellow, dreamy, introspective

Cultural Association: Jazz, pop music, folk music

G Lydian Scale: G, A, B, C#, D, E, F#

Emotions: Dreamy, uplifting, mystical

Cultural Association: Jazz, pop music, progressive rock

G Mixolydian Scale: G, A, B, C, D, E, F

Emotions: Groovy, bluesy, uplifting

Cultural Association: Rock music, blues, funk

<u>G#</u>

G# Major Scale - G#, A#, C, C#, D#, F, G - majestic, grand, triumphant, bold

G# Minor Scale - G#, A#, B, C#, D#, E, F# - intense, dramatic, melancholy, sad, tragic

G# Harmonic Minor Scale - G#, A#, B, C#, D#, E, G -

exotic, dark, mysterious, dramatic

G# Phrygian Dominant Scale - G#, A, B, C#, D#, E, F - intense, exotic, mysterious, fiery

G# Whole Tone Scale - G#, A#, C, D, D#, F - dreamy, ethereal, mysterious, otherworldly

A

A Major Scale - A, B, C#, D, E, F#, G# - bright, joyful, happy, triumphant

A Minor Scale - A, B, C, D, E, F, G - dark, somber, melancholy, introspective, yearning

A Dorian Scale - A, B, C, D, E, F#, G - jazzy, mellow, relaxed

A Mixolydian Scale - A, B, C#, D, E, F#, G - bluesy, funky, upbeat, adventurous

A Phrygian Scale - A, A#, C, D, E, F, G - exotic, mysterious, intense, passionate

A#

A# Major Scale - A#, C, D, D#, F, G, A - majestic, grand, triumphant, bold

A# Minor Scale - A#, B, C#, D#, E, F#, G# - intense, dramatic, melancholy, sad, tragic

A# Harmonic Minor Scale - A#, B, C#, D#, E, F#, A - exotic, dark, mysterious, dramatic

A# Phrygian Dominant Scale - A#, B, C#, D#, E, F#,

G - intense, exotic, mysterious, fiery

A# Whole Tone Scale - A#, C, D, E, F#, G# - dreamy, ethereal, mysterious, otherworldly

<u>B</u>

B Major Scale - B, C#, D#, E, F#, G#, A# - bright, joyful, happy, triumphant

B Minor Scale - B, C#, D, E, F#, G, A - dark, somber, melancholy, introspective, yearning

B Dorian Scale - B, C#, D, E, F#, G#, A - jazzy, mellow, relaxed

B Mixolydian Scale - B, C#, D#, E, F#, G#, A - bluesy, funky, upbeat, adventurous

B Phrygian Scale - B, C, D, E, F#, G, A - exotic, mysterious, intense, passionate

Keep in mind that each of these scales was converted to be able to pick and play with Alchemy bowls™.

Singing Bowls with World Melodies

As a bonus. I wanted to take melodies and adapt them for Singing Bowls.

I'm only providing 1 song for the first 3 below as well as Durin's song as a fan favorite but considering the list of world melodies below feel free to look up any of those categories, find songs and create your own adaptations.

1. Lullabies
2. Hymns
3. Folk Songs
4. Ballads
5. Anthems
6. Sea Shanties
7. Nursery Rhymes
8. Acoustic Serenades
9. Spirituals
10. Drinking Songs
11. Dirges
12. Chants
13. Warsongs
14. Miscellaneous
15. Etc

The choice to use a relatively small number of notes in the adaptations provided here, such as 9 notes rather than 20 or 30+, is driven by a few considerations.

Fewer notes make the adaptations more accessible to a wider range of participants, regardless of their musical background or experience with singing Bowls. It allows individuals to engage with the practice more easily. One of the primary purposes of using singing Bowls is to facilitate meditation, reflection, and contemplation.

A simpler melody line helps maintain a meditative atmosphere without overwhelming the practitioner or listener with complex musical arrangements. Singing bowls, while capable of producing rich and resonant tones, have certain limitations in terms of pitch range and the ease of playing rapid successions of notes or complex melodies.

The beauty of singing bowls lies in their rich overtones and the resonance of each strike. Fewer notes allow each struck note to resonate fully, creating a space for the overtones to be heard and appreciated. Most people will also not own 20-30 Bowls or be able to play more than 2 at a time. The Notes selected for the songs I listed are. C4

- D4
- E4
- F4
- G4
- A4
- B4
- C5
- D5
- E5

This was easy to do because all of the singing bowls fall within this range but feel free to change the notes or scale depending on your musical taste.

Also, When trying to figure out exactly how to play these with bowls and what parts to sing on what note exactly this isn't intended to be like reading music sheets and that's on purpose. I want people to be creative and adapt it to how it suits them based on their intuition, vocal range, the way they play and their creativity. But for some guidance I do provide simple instructions.

Lullabies

Lullabies are among one of the the most ancient forms of musical expression, serving to soothe infants and aid in sleep.

These songs are characterized by their soft melodies and rhythmic simplicity, often accompanied by gentle, rocking motions. They exist in every culture and are usually among the first forms of music that children are exposed to.The oldest known lullaby dates back to about 2000 BC, found on a clay tablet in Babylon and was left with a charm. This Included a plea to the gods to protect the child. In Greek mythology, the goddess Hera sent Hypnos, the personification of sleep, to lull Zeus to sleep with a song, showcasing the use of lullabies in various texts across time.

Brahms' Lullaby *(Wiegenlied: Guten Abend, gute Nacht)*

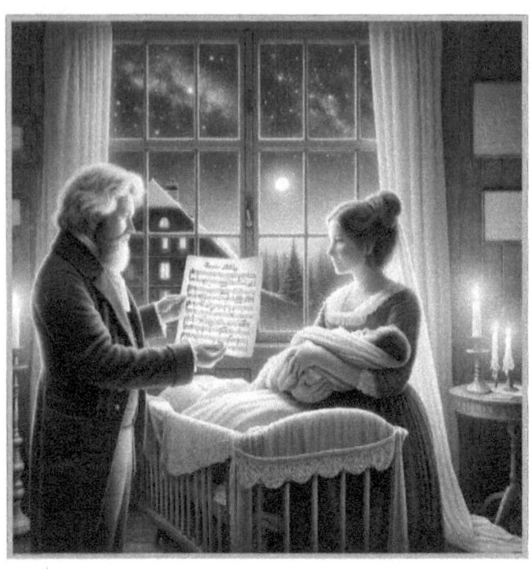

Origin: **Germany**

Johannes Brahms's "Wiegenlied: Guten Abend, gute Nacht," universally known as "Brahms' Lullaby," Composed in 1868, this iconic lullaby was Brahms's gift to Bertha Faber, a dear friend from his childhood, to celebrate the birth of her second son, Hans. The melody was inspired by a song Bertha herself used to sing, drawing from a Silesian folk tune that Brahms transformed into a symbol of maternal love and care.

"Good evening, good night,"

    Melody: C4 (Good) - E4 (eve-) - G4 (-ning,) | C5 (good) - G4 (night,)

    (Pause)

"Adorned with roses,"

> Melody: E4 (A-) - G4 (dorned) - C5 (with) - G4 (roses,)
>
> (Pause)

"With carnations covered,"

> Melody: E4 (With) - G4 (car-) - C5 (-na-) - G4 (tions) | C5 (cov-) - G4 (-ered,)
>
> (Pause)

"Slip under the blanket:"

> Melody: C4 (Slip) - E4 (un-) - G4 (der) | G4 (the) - E4 (blan-) - C4 (ket,)
>
> (Pause)

"Tomorrow morning, if God wills,"

> Melody: C4 (To-) - D4 (mor-) - E4 (row) | E4 (morn-) - G4 (ing,) | C4 (if) - G4 (God) - E4 (wills,)
>
> (Pause)

"You will be awakened again."

> Melody: C4 (You) - D4 (will) - E4 (be) | G4 (a-) - E4 (wak-) - C4 (ened) | G4 (a-) - E4 (gain.)
>
> (Pause)

"Good evening, good night," (repeated with same melody as the first line of the first stanza)

> Melody: C4 (Good) - E4 (eve-) - G4 (-ning,) | C5 (good) - G4 (night,)
>
> (Pause)

"Watched over by little angels,"

> Melody: E4 (Watch-) - G4 (ed) - C5 (o-) | C5 (ver) - G4 (by) - E4 (lit-) - G4 (tle) - E4 (an-) - G4 (gels,)
> (Pause)

"They show in your dream,"

> Melody: E4 (They) - G4 (show) - C5 (in) - G4 (your) - E4 (dream,)
> (Pause)

"The Christ-child's tree:"

> Melody: C4 (The) - E4 (Christ-) - G4 (child's) - C5 (tree,)
> (Pause)

"Sleep now blissfully and sweetly,"

> Melody: C4 (Sleep) - D4 (now) - E4 (bliss-) | G4 (ful-) - E4 (ly) - C4 (and) | G4 (sweet-) - E4 (ly,)
> (Pause)

"See paradise in your dream."

> Melody: C4 (See) - D4 (par-) - E4 (a-) - G4 (dise) | E4 (in) - C4 (your) - G4 (dream.)
> (Pause)

Hymns

Hymns are spiritual songs that express religious belief and are used in worship. With roots tracing back to ancient civilizations, hymns were initially part of the Sumerian and Greek religious practices, evolving significantly in the Christian tradition. Many hymns in ancient cultures were dedicated to deities. The Rig Veda, a sacred Indian collection, includes hymns praising the pantheon of Vedic gods, showing the connection between music, the divine, and the cosmos.

Raghupati Raghav Raja Ram

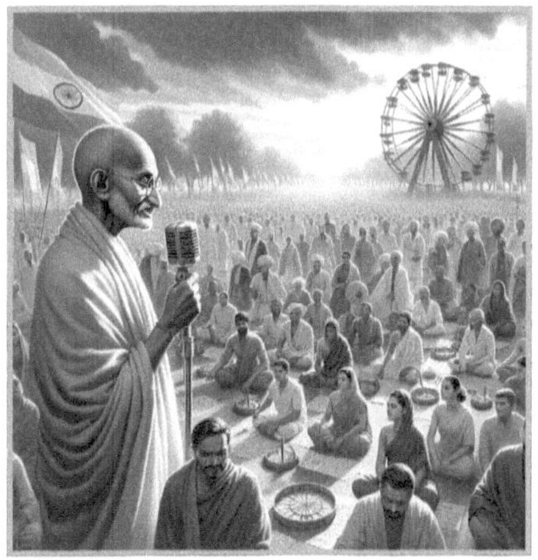

Origin: *India*
Religion: *Hinduism*

Gandhi, who led India to independence through non-violent resistance, often used this song to promote peace, unity, and the moral strength of nonviolence. The hymn praises Lord Rama, an avatar of Vishnu, embodying the virtues of righteousness, justice, and the protection of the weak. The inclusion of the line "Ishwar Allah Tero Naam," calling upon both Hindu and Muslim names for the divine, underscores Gandhi's commitment to religious harmony. This bhajan not only strengthened the resolve of those fighting for India's freedom but also conveyed a powerful message of inclusivity and faith in the divine.

"Lord Rama, the chief of the house of Raghu, Uplifter of the fallen, with Sita"

Melody: C4 (Lord) - D4 (Ra-) - E4 (ma,) | F4 (the) - G4 (chief) - A4 (of) - G4 (the) - F4 (house,) | E4 (of) - D4 (Rag-) - C4 (hu,) | C4 (Up-) - D4 (lift-) - E4 (er) - F4 (of) - G4 (the) - A4 (fall-) - G4 (en,) | F4 (with) - E4 (Si-)) - D4 (ta)

(Pause)

"Beautiful Vibhishana and Pavana worship Sita and Rama, Oh dear, worship Sita and Rama"

Melody: G4 (Beau-) - A4 (ti-) - B4 (ful) | C5 (Vib-) - D5 (hish-) - E5 (an-) | A4 (and) - B4 (Pav-) - C5 (an-) - D5 (a) | G4 (wor-) - A4 (ship) | B4 (Si-) - C5 (ta) - D5 (and) - E5 (Ra-) - C5 (ma,) | G4 (Oh) - A4 (dear,) | B4 (wor-)

- C5 (ship) - D5 (Si-) - E5 (ta) - D5 (and) - C5 (Ra-) - B4 (ma)

(Pause)

"God or Allah is your name, Lord, give wisdom to all"
Melody: E4 (God) - F4 (or) - G4 (Al-) - A4 (lah) | G4 (is) - F4 (your) - E4 (name,) | A4 (Lord,) - G4 (give) - F4 (wis-) - E4 (dom) | A4 (to) - G4 (all)
(Pause)

Begin with a foundational drone on C4, creating a tranquil backdrop. Integrate drones on G4 or E4 to highlight emotional or pivotal moments in the hymn, enriching the auditory experience and the devotional atmosphere.

Folk Songs

Folk songs often cover a wide range of topics, from work and love to politics and humor, reflecting the everyday lives of people. The English folk song "Greensleeves" dates back to the 16th century and has endured in popularity, evolving in lyrics and melody over centuries. Its origins are shrouded in myth. Many folk songs are steeped in legend, such as the Scottish "Tam Lin," which tells of a young woman rescuing her lover from the Fairy Queen, highlighting the blend of realistic emotion and mythical storytelling.

Scarborough Fair

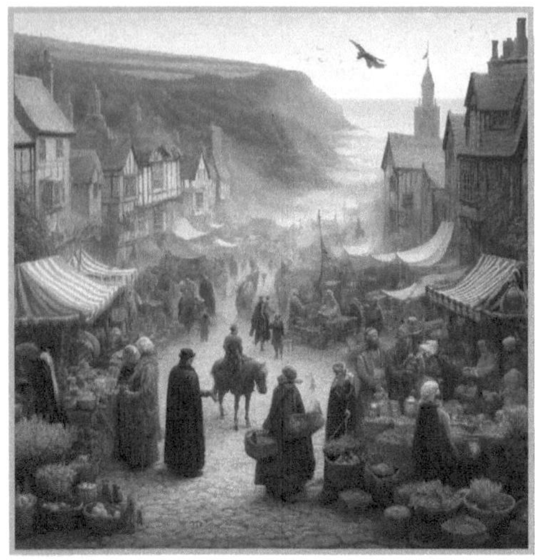

Origin: *England*

"Scarborough Fair," a traditional English ballad, carries the fragrance of the Late Middle Ages through its verses, speaking of love, herbal emblems, and quests for the unattainable. It became particularly resonant during the Scarborough Fair in Yorkshire, a grand 45-day event that was a hub for merchants across England. The song was later popularized by Simon & Garfunkel, thus moving it into the fabric of modern musical heritage. It's a narrative that bridges the medieval with the contemporary.

"Are you going to Scarborough Fair? Parsley, sage, rosemary, and thyme."

Melody: C4 - D4 - E4 (Are you going) | F4 - G4 - A4 (to Scarborough) | B4 - C5 (Fair?) | G4 - F4 - E4 - D4 (Parsley, sage, rosemary,) | C4 (and thyme.)
(Pause)

"Remember me to one who lives there, for once she was a true love of mine."

Melody: C5 - B4 - A4 (Remember me to one) | G4 - F4 - E4 (who lives there,) | D4 - C4 (for once she was) | F4 - E4 - D4 - C4 (a true love of mine.)
(Pause)

"Tell her to make me a cambric shirt, parsley, sage, rosemary, and thyme."

Melody: D4 - E4 - F4 (Tell her to make me) | G4 - A4 - B4 (a cambric shirt,) | C5 - D5 (parsley, sage,) | B4 - A4 - G4 - F4 (rosemary, and thyme.)
(Pause)

"Without no seams nor needlework, then she'll be a true love of mine."

Melody: D5 - C5 - B4 (Without no seams) | A4 - G4 - F4 (nor needlework,) | E4 - D4 (then she'll be) | F4 - E4 - D4 - C4 (a true love of mine.)
(Pause)

"Tell her to find me an acre of land, parsley, sage, rosemary, and thyme."

Melody: E4 - F4 - G4 (Tell her to find me) | A4 - B4 - C5 (an acre of land,) | D5 - E5 (parsley, sage,) | C5 - B4 - A4 - G4 (rosemary, and thyme.)

(Pause)

"Between the salt water and the sea strands, then she'll be a true love of mine."

Melody: E5 - D5 - C5 (Between the salt water) | B4 - A4 - G4 (and the sea strands,) | F4 - E4 (then she'll be) | G4 - F4 - E4 - D4 (a true love of mine.)

(Pause)

Harmony/Drones: A drone on C4 underpins the melody, offering a steady tonal backdrop

Bonus

Durin's Song

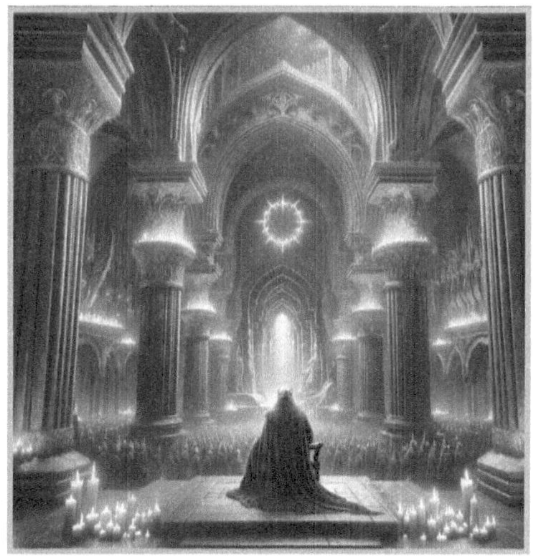

Origin: *Middle-earth (Fantasy)*

"Durin's Song" is of Dwarven lore within J.R.R. Tolkien's Middle-earth, the saga of Durin, one of the original Seven Fathers of the Dwarves. This ballad tells of Durin's awakening and his establishment of the mightiest Dwarven kingdom, Khazad-dûm, known in its decline as Moria. Evoking the majesty of the Dwarven halls and the beauty of their fading glory.

"The world was young, the mountains green, No stain yet

on the Moon was seen."

>Melody: C4 (The) - D4 (world) - E4 (was young,) | F4 (the moun-) - G4 (tains green,) | A4 (No stain) - G4 (yet) - F4 (on the) - E4 (Moon was seen.)
>(Pause)

"No words were laid on stream or stone, When Durin woke and walked alone."

>Melody: E4 (No words) - F4 (were laid) - G4 (on stream) | A4 (or stone,) | B4 (When Du-) - A4 (rin woke) - G4 (and walked) - F4 (alone.)
>(Pause)

"He named the nameless hills and dells; He drank from yet untasted wells."

>Melody: G4 (He named) - A4 (the name-) - B4 (less hills) | C5 (and dells;) | D5 (He drank) - C5 (from yet) - B4 (untasted) - A4 (wells.)
>(Pause)

"He stooped and looked in Mirrormere, And saw a crown of stars appear,"

>Melody: A4 (He stooped) - G4 (and looked) - F4 (in Mirror-) - E4 (mere,) | D4 (And saw) - C4 (a crown) - D4 (of stars) - E4 (appear,)
>(Pause)

"As gems upon a silver thread, Above the shadows of his head."

Melody: F4 (As gems) - G4 (upon a) - A4 (silver) - B4 (thread,) | C5 (Above the) - D5 (shadows) - C5 (of his) - B4 (head.)

(Pause)

HOW TO PLAY A CRYSTAL BOWL

While there are numerous resources like books and YouTube tutorials available on playing singing bowls, there's still a need for a concise guide to address common mistakes and misconceptions. This short guide focuses on playing Crystal bowls, as techniques may vary for Tibetan bowls and others.

Step One: Purposeful Playing

Begin by understanding why you are playing the alchemy bowl. Whether it's for meditation, healing, breathwork etc, clarity on your intention is always important.

Step Two: Mindful Approach

Crystal bowls are crafted from crystal, distinct from metal bowls. Avoid the misconception that they can be played with the same force. Unlike metal bowls, crystal bowls are fragile. Treat them delicately, avoiding forceful banging. While frosted crystal bowls allow for more assertive playing, remember the general rule is to handle them with care.

"Force may clear a path, but a garden truly flourishes when cultivated with patience, understanding, and mutual respect."

Individuality of Bowls

Each crystal bowl is unique, resonating at its specific frequency. Some bowls may respond differently to playing techniques. External factors like temperature and the energy of the person playing can influence the sound. Treat each bowl with respect, understanding that the energy you bring to playing it impacts the outcome.

Avoid Playing Inside the Bowl

A common mistake is attempting to play singing bowls on the inside. Stick to playing on the exterior for the best results.

Equipment: Mallet

To play a singing bowl, you'll need a suitable mallet. Ensure you have the right tool for the job to produce the desired sound without causing damage. Some people argue over which mallet is best. I've seen everything from what crystal tones® and other companies use to people at a park in Portland using sticks with leaves and crystals attached that were still able to get amazing sounds out of the bowls. Play around with the different mallets and then master whichever one feels the most comfortable to you and your technique.

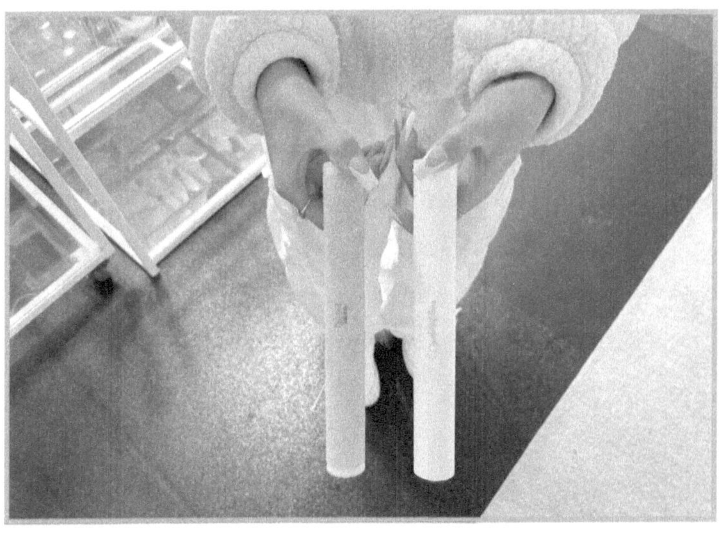

Crystal Tones® Mallets for Alchemy Bowls™

Crystal Tones® offers two popular types of mallets for playing Alchemy Bowls™: Suede Mallets (on the left) and Sonic Mallets (on the right). While I won't list all the mallets or Crystal Tones® products here, you can explore their complete inventory on the Crystal Tones® website.

1. Suede Mallets (on the left):

- Preferred by early adopters, Crystal Tones'® top partners, and those who play on the side of the bowl instead of around the rim.

- When used around the rim, the suede produces a sandpaper-like noise, but when played on the side, it glides effortlessly.
- Note: Suede mallets are not vegan-friendly.

2. Sonic Mallets (on the right):

- A newer option and a personal favorite for many.
- There is no definitive "better" or "worse" choice; it depends on your playing style. Instruments are unique, and people play them differently.
- Sonic mallets have gained popularity since their release and are typically sent by Crystal Tones® when someone purchases a bowl unless suede is specifically requested.
- When playing around the rim, sonic mallets do not produce noise, providing a simpler playing experience.

Remember, choosing between suede and sonic mallets is a matter of personal preference and playing style.

Additional Tool: 0-Ring:

- In addition to the mallet, you'll need a 0-ring.

For a comprehensive view of Crystal Tones'® mallets and other products, visit their official website. This information is tailored specifically for Alchemy Bowls™, and the website provides a broader overview of their offerings.

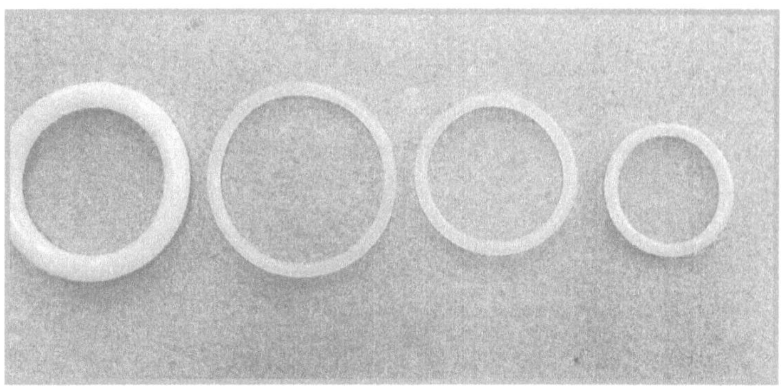

When playing a singing bowl, you have the option to play it in your hand or on a hard surface. Using an O-ring, however, enhances the experience by preventing tipping and minimizing sound interference on surfaces like carpet. Different O-ring sizes are available to accommodate various bowl sizes:

- Smallest O-Ring: Designed for 6-inch bowls.
- Medium O-Ring: Suitable for 7-9 inch bowls.
- Large O-Ring: Intended for 10 inches and larger bowls.
- Thicker Donut Ring (far left): Specifically for bowls with a round bottom instead of a flat one.

Playing Technique:

Hold the Mallet Like a Pencil:
- Start by holding the mallet in a manner similar to

holding a pencil. This provides control and precision in your movements.

Initiating Sound:

- There are two initial methods to produce sound:
- Light Chiming: Hold the mallet lightly and gently chime the bowl to initiate sound. This is a basic technique suitable for beginners.
- Gliding: Do not chime and just Start by gliding the mallet around the rim of the bowl until the sound picks up. As you progress, explore more advanced techniques for nuanced and varied sounds.

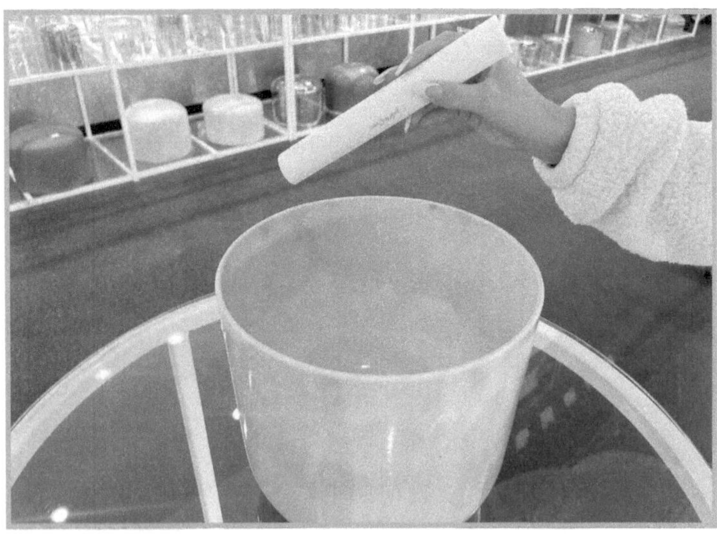

Remember, the O-ring helps stabilize the bowl during play, making it easier to produce consistent and clear sounds.

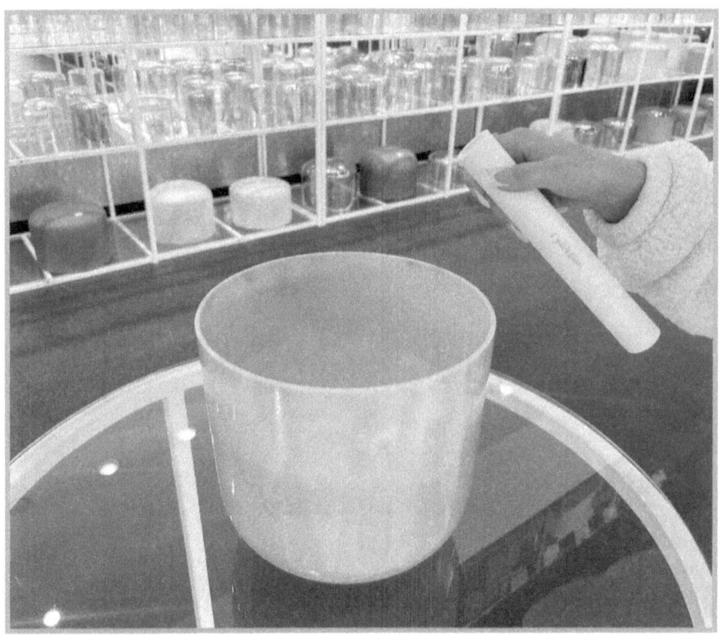

Once you have initiated the sound, the next step is to refine it by gently gliding the mallet around the bowl.

Mallet Glide Technique:

- Hold the mallet with the same precision as before and glide it around the bowl , neither too heavy nor too light.

Avoid Excessive Pressure:

- Applying too much pressure may muffle the sound, while too little can cause the mallet to bounce off, resulting in an unpleasant noise. Find the right balance to maintain a clear and resonant tone.

Moderate Pace:

- Move the mallet around the bowl at a moderate pace. Not too fast, not too slow. The goal is to coax the bowl into revealing its unique sound.

Let the Bowl Sing:

- Once the bowl begins to produce its song, you have the option to either step back and let it sing out on its own or to continue stabilizing the sound.

Listen for Feedback:

- Pay close attention to the sound produced. If the bowl starts buzzing or creating an unpleasant noise, it indicates a need for adjustment in pressure or pace.

Caution against Forceful Pace:

- Be cautious not to continue at a forceful pace if the bowl is producing an unpleasant sound. Vibrations bouncing inside the bowl can lead to shattering. Take heed of any signs of strain in the sound.

Remember, the key is to listen to the bowl and adjust your technique. A mindful and patient approach will allow the bowl to resonate freely, creating harmony.

Overtones and Undertones in Singing bowls: An important consideration in playing Bowls is the choice between chiming the bowl Chapter 7: Crating sets 309 initially or starting directly with rim play. Here's why skipping the chime and diving into rim play can offer unique benefits:

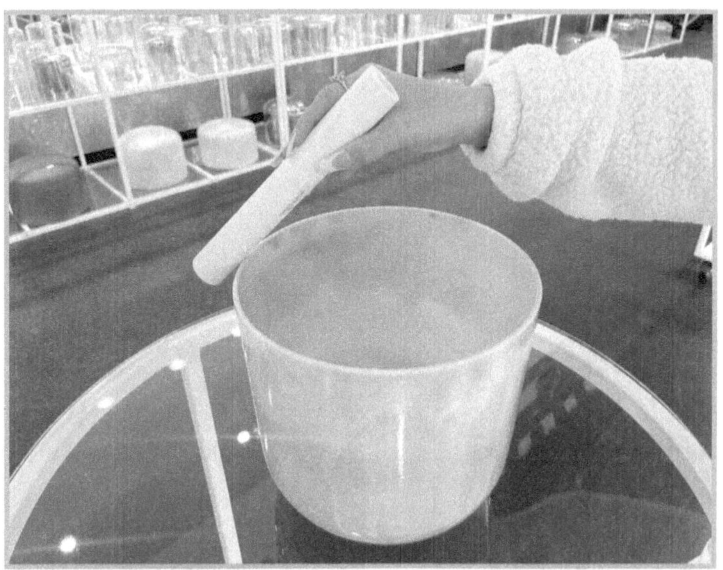

Overtones and Undertones:

- Chiming the bowl produces overtones, but when you move to rim play, you can explore more pronounced undertones. This choice allows you to decide whether you prefer a combination of both or a more focused emphasis on one.

Intentional Playing:

- Consider your intention – do you want a transitional, wind-like flow between bowls during a session, or do you prefer a more activating experience by chiming each bowl? The decision should align with your purpose, making each session intentional and meaningful.

Graceful Transitions:
- Opting for direct rim play enables seamless transitions between bowls, creating a graceful and continuous sound without the need for individual chimes.

Side Playing - The Violin or Eastern Approach:
An alternative technique is the "violin" or Eastern way of playing, which involves rubbing the bowl on the side. This method offers a nuanced range of tones:

Lower Tones (Rubbing Towards the Bottom):
- Rubbing the bowl on the side towards the bottom produces lower tones.

This technique can be used to evoke a deep resonance from the bowl.

Higher Tones (Rubbing Higher Up):
- Moving higher up on the side produces higher tones. With skillful practice, you can isolate and play with these higher frequencies, creating a dynamic and varied experience.

Advanced Octave Changes:

- Some bowls can shift octaves based on the rubbing location. For instance, a bowl may start as a 3rd or 4th octave A when rubbed lower on the side, transitioning to a 5th octave D# when played around the rim. This advanced technique requires practice and precision.

In summary, the decision to chime or not and the exploration of different playing techniques depend on your intention and the experience you want to create.

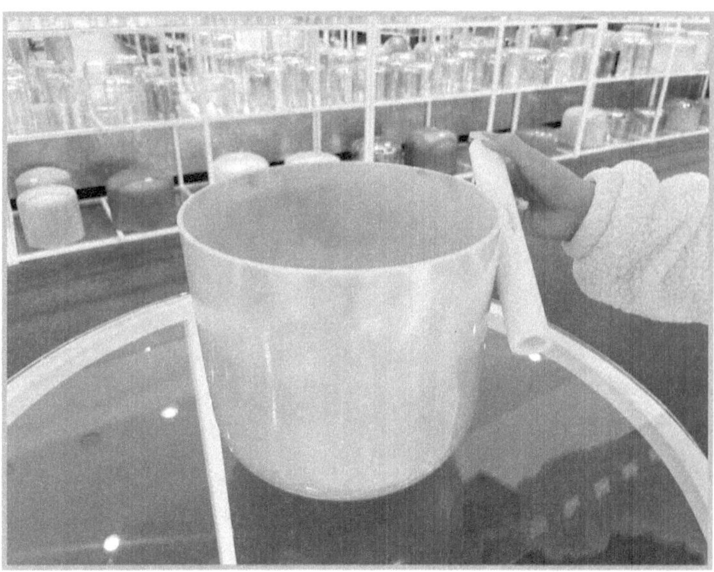

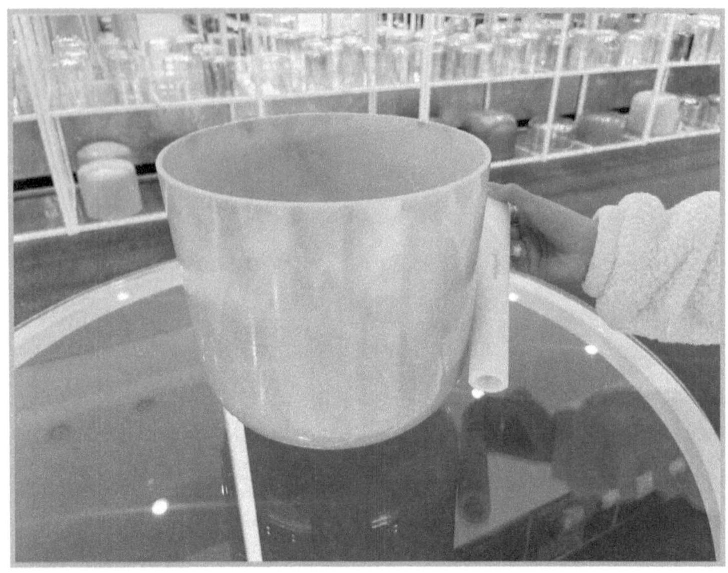

Chapter 8

SAFETY, CONSENT, AND POST-SESSION SUPPORT

MY FIRST SOUND BATH

My first sound bath/session happened 5-6 months after I was hired by Crystal Tones®. Most of my job up until that point had been hands-on learning, building sets, research, developing systems, answering emails, fulfilling orders, and working to improve things within the company.

Crystal Tones® was mainly closed to the public, and the partners who came by to pick up bowls were usually on a limited time frame, focused solely on getting their work done. As a result, I had yet to have the opportunity to do any sound baths for anyone. When we went to Tucson, Arizona, for the yearly gem show for the company, I was thrown into demonstrations and being hands-on with customers.

One of the days we were working, an older lady

appeared outside the tent, initially refusing to enter. She seemed distressed and apprehensive; her energy was heavy. Under her breath and almost fearful, she started talking about the mistakes she had made in her life and the choices she regretted. She believed that she was paying for her past actions and was going through a difficult period because of them, both emotionally and financially.

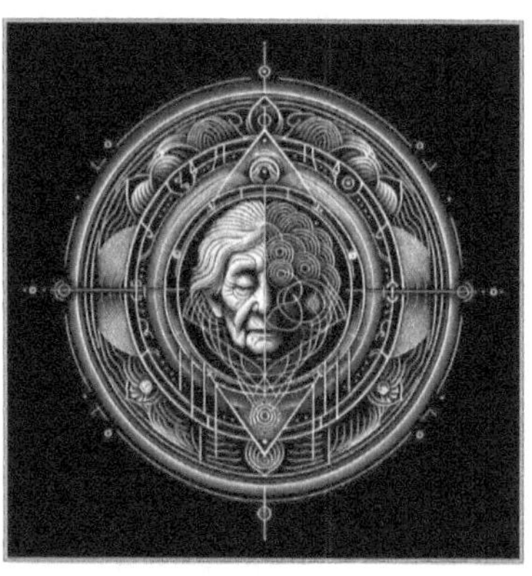

She asked if we would give her a sound healing session. While I didn't want to turn her down, I also didn't want to offer something that I had never entirely done before. Fortunately another employee with experience in sound healing offered to help.

We set up a space in the middle of the tent for the lady. The other employee began playing selected bowls and guided the lady through a meditation on letting go of old patterns. Meanwhile, I used a hand practitioner and guided the bowl over her body, intending to bring peace.

During this, I had an intuitive moment where I asked in my mind if we could release her from her trauma and karma to do so.

At the same time, the lady's breathing became abnormal, and her entire body started shaking. My coworker continued playing with the bowls and placed their hand on her forehead, encouraging her to let go. This process lasted several minutes.

Eventually, she settled down and was guided out of the sound bath. As she sat up, she appeared to be a different person. She smiled, made eye contact, and discussed her life goals and plans. She even confessed her involvement in black magic in the past and how she used to manipulate energy to harm others and has had a hard time repaying those debts but felt like the sound bath we gave her even if it only lasted 10-15 minutes helped her to break through some of those paradigms.

When I returned to Tucson the following year, I unexpectedly reencountered her, and she was wearing bright colors. She looked genuinely happy, positive energy, She remembered and warmly hugged me, expressing her gratitude for the changes in her life.

That initial encounter forced me to reevaluate, sparking a pursuit of further learning. The responsibility of healing through sound is overlooked. It can be portrayed on social media as a vibrant tapestry of colors, idyllic retreats, impressive results, and carefully curated highlight reels.

Even when glimpses of people releasing their pain are shared, it often appears glamorous, accompanied by uplifting music. I've even been guilty of portraying it this way to make it seem more inviting.

However, that first experience felt more like an exorcism. The sounds she emitted, the dry labored breathing, choking on her words, the convulsions. I had no clue how to handle the situation if it worsened. It made me realize that people sometimes perceive sound healing as a passing trend, overlooking the true essence of being a healer. To be a healer means working with individuals who need and seek healing. And if someone requires healing, it signifies something is fundamentally wrong — an issue that must be confronted and wrestled with. This can be messy. Any aspiring healer must decide how far they are willing to venture into to provide guidance and support to those seeking help.

Mount Shasta

Shortly after my return from Tucson, the company approached me with an intriguing proposal: relocating to Mount Shasta, California, to assist in the opening and managing of a Crystal Tones® retail store. My intuition strongly urged me to embrace this opportunity, as I had spent years researching Mount Shasta, Telos, Adama, Ufos, St Germain, and all the other Shasta stories. Yet, it always seemed to elude me. Sound baths would likely be a significant part of our offerings in this new location. During the drive down, I vividly remember immersing myself in various books on sound healing, with Sarah Auster's work as one of my favorites as well as Jay emmanuel.

Fast forward to my time in Shasta, I was trying to integrate into the community and host sound baths. One of the earliest experiences involved myself and one of our employees, conducting an individual sound bath for a tourist who had traveled from overseas to explore the beauty of Shasta.

We set the stage, surrounding the person with various bowls, including a few 16-inch SuperGrades™. We had a specific chord in mind, incorporating binaural elements and setting intentions for the session.

The sound bath lasted approximately 45 minutes. As we approached the conclusion of the sound bath, I recall my coworker gently instructing the individual to sit up. However, I had a lingering feeling that we were rushing them or that it was too soon. It wasn't their fault, but it seemed evident that the person was still transitioning, not fully present or grounded.

Even when they managed to rise and reach the door to leave, it was apparent that they struggled to string together coherent sentences. I felt uneasy about letting them go in that state. It became another realization for me—an awakening to the fact that, although I was educated with the building of sets and felt comfortable playing the bowls and sharing my knowledge, I had failed to consider the importance of aftercare. I hadn't considered what the individual might be going through or dealing with immediately following the sound bath or even in the following days. How long did the residual effects last? How long did shifts continue to occur within them? These questions weighed heavily on my mind as I recognized the significance of providing proper support and guidance beyond the session.

Energy

In addition to my revelations regarding aftercare, I also began noticing a pattern. After certain sound baths, I found myself utterly exhausted. I would invest considerable time and effort into constructing intentional sets and meticulously arranging the space. I approached each session carefully and made sure that I was curating an experience based on questions that I would ask the client or a group of people, depending on whether it would just be a general or a specialized session. But I wasn't just tired; I felt drained and depleted afterward.

While I acknowledge the numerous theories and that certain practitioners possess higher intuition, expertise, and practice in this field, I can only share my personal experience and insights.

One theory that resonates with me is that exhaustion arises when one leads with ego, believing they are responsible for the healing process as if they are the source: their skill, their time, their energy. This mindset can deplete one's life force energy, as they draw from their personal energy pool to fuel the healing sessions, The intentions here can play a part too. Are you really in service or are you trying to get them to buy bowls or book further sessions.

In contrast, an alternative philosophy suggests that healing energy is inherent in the fundamental state of the universe, with an infinite supply of chi, prana, and life force available.

As a healer, one can become a conduit, a medium through which this energy and intention flows. In this perspective, it is not the healer's personal energy utilized but rather the intentional and universal energies that pass through them. They act as a channel, facilitating the flow.

When I began to adopt this perspective and practice, I noticed a significant shift. Instead of feeling depleted, I felt empowered and energized. Recognizing myself as a vessel through which healing energy flows. 40 minutes could pass and it only felt like ten. Of course, these insights are specific to my journey and experience.

Some healers do meditations first to cover themselves in protective white light so they don't absorb any of the energies possibly being released. There are lots of protection meditations you could just look up online if interested.

Some sound baths focus solely on singing bowls, while others incorporate a variety of instruments such as gongs, chimes, drums, or even vocal toning. Additionally, practitioners may enhance the experience by setting up a crystal grid or utilizing essential oils and incense to create an immersive atmosphere. Sound baths can cater to different scales, ranging from grand events with thousands of participants to intimate sessions designed for a single individual.

As you embark on your sound healing journey, you should pause and reflect on various aspects that will shape your path. Asking yourself a series of questions can help clarify your intentions and guide your decisions.

Direction

Firstly, consider what you truly want to achieve through sound healing. Are you aiming to provide a healing experience, facilitate relaxation and stress relief, or explore the intersection of sound and spirituality? It could be activation, an ecstatic dance-type experience. Defining your purpose will help you cultivate a clear vision and set a direction for your practice.

Next, consider your target audience or the participants you want to attract. Are you interested in working with individuals seeking emotional healing, such as those in need of rehabilitation, domestic violence victims, or people who have been sex trafficked?

Are you focused on individuals seeking physical rejuvenation, similar to those who require physical therapy? Perhaps your intended audience consists of individuals who have sustained physical injuries and need specialized care and rehabilitation.

Alternatively, do you cater to those seeking spiritual growth, individuals who have a desire to connect with angels, access higher vibrational states, or explore their spiritual journey?

The list goes on, but by identifying your ideal audience, you can tailor your offerings and create an environment that resonates with their needs and the future version of your practice.

Exploring instruments is another step. Which instruments resonate with you the most? Are you captivated by the ethereal tones of singing bowls, the primal rhythms of drums, or the expansive vibrations of gongs? Focusing on specific instruments allows you to develop expertise and deepen your connection to their unique healing properties.

Consider the desired takeaways you wish to offer your clients. What do you want them to experience or gain from the sound bath? Clarifying the outcomes you aim to facilitate will help shape the structure and intention of your sessions.

Pricing is another aspect to consider. What is your value on your time, energy, and expertise? How much will you charge for your sound bath sessions? Researching industry standards, considering your level of experience, and evaluating the market demand will aid in determining an appropriate pricing structure.

Lastly, reflect on any internal or external obstacles that might be hindering your progress. What

fears, self-doubt, or limiting beliefs holding you back from fully embracing your path as a sound healer? Are there practical challenges, such as finding suitable venues, acquiring instruments, or establishing a client base? Identifying these barriers allows you to devise strategies to overcome them and confidently move forward. Trust your intuition, pay for mentors, embrace the process, read, play and allow your passion for sound healing to guide you toward a fulfilling and impactful practice.

Clear Intention

Clear intention and creating a safe space where individuals can feel comfortable. One of the aspects of facilitating a successful session is to not bring your own personal issues or emotional baggage into the experience. This is vital because many people may not be receptive if they detect that your energy is "off." Are you an embodiment of the principles you teach? Participants will be more receptive if they perceive that you authentically embody the teachings and practices you advocate. Nobody's perfect, but you are at least on the journey. Being the result of your teaching means demonstrating the positive effects of the principles and techniques you share. Yes, we can learn something from everyone and have creative and wholesome takeaways, but considering if you are yourself even on the path of what you are trying to sell people on or provide is huge.

BARRIERS

So many people unknowingly live in a defensive state, trapped within a pattern shaped by their experiences in the world. Each day, we can encounter disharmony and conflicts. People perceive us in specific ways, and those in positions of authority—be it bosses, coworkers, or friends—address us in particular manners. Our trust in things may be shattered with time, leaving us guarded and cautious.

The rise of social media has only amplified these challenges, making it even more challenging for healers to navigate through the noise. As a sound healer, your role is to transcend everyone else's conventional modes of communication. This is where the power of music and sound emerges as something truly remarkable. Regardless of who you are, where you come from, or your race, certain sounds and melodies can unlock people's hearts and liberate their emotions. Music and sound provide a gateway to authenticity and vulnerability in a world often clouded by Walls built to protect but as a consequence could also be holding you back from becoming the most authentic version of yourself.

PRECAUTIONS

While sound baths and vibrational therapy are generally considered safe and beneficial for many individuals, there are some cases where caution or avoidance may be necessary. It is important to note that the following list is not exhaustive, and it is always recommended to consult with a qualified healthcare professional before engaging in any alternative therapies, especially if you have pre-existing medical conditions.

Here are some examples of individuals who should

exercise caution or avoid sound baths and vibrational therapy:

Pregnant women: Some specific frequencies or vibrations may not be suitable during pregnancy, especially in the first trimester. It is essential to consult with a healthcare provider before engaging in sound baths or vibrational therapy.

Individuals with epilepsy or seizure disorders: Certain sound frequencies or intense vibrations may potentially trigger seizures in susceptible individuals. Those with epilepsy or seizure disorders should proceed cautiously and consult their healthcare provider.

People with heart conditions: Intense vibrations or loud sounds may impact heart rhythm or blood pressure. Individuals with heart conditions, such as arrhythmias or high blood pressure should consult their healthcare provider before participating in sound baths or vibrational therapy.

Individuals with implanted medical devices: Some sound therapy techniques involve using powerful vibrations or magnetic fields, which could interfere with implanted medical devices like pacemakers or cochlear implants. It is crucial to consult with a healthcare professional and follow their guidance.

People with recent surgeries or injuries: Vibrations and specific frequencies may interfere with the healing process of fresh surgical incisions or wounds. It is advisable to wait until the recovery period is over and receive clearance from a healthcare provider before undergoing sound baths or vibrational therapy.

Those with active infections or contagious diseases: In some cases, sound baths may involve group settings where individuals share the same space. If you have an active infection or a contagious condition, it is considerate to avoid attending sound bath sessions to prevent the spread of illness to others.

Individuals with severe mental health conditions: Sound baths can induce deep relaxation and altered states of consciousness. While this can be beneficial for many people, individuals with extreme mental health conditions such as schizophrenia or dissociative disorders should approach these therapies with caution and seek guidance from mental health professionals.

Children and infants: Sound baths and vibrational therapy may not be suitable for young children or infants due to their delicate sensory systems. It is advisable to consult with a pediatrician or healthcare provider before exposing young children to these therapies.

Individuals with sensitive hearing or sound sensitivity disorders: Some people have heightened sensitivity to sound, known as hyperacusis or misophonia. In such cases, specific frequencies or intense sounds used in sound baths may be overwhelming or distressing. It is recommended to proceed cautiously and adjust the intensity or duration of exposure as needed.

People with acute medical conditions: If an individual is experiencing a sudden medical emergency, it is essential to prioritize appropriate medical care rather than engaging in sound baths or vibrational therapy. Seek immediate medical attention in such situations.

A few specific types of medical implants could be affected by sound baths and may make them less optimal or require caution.The implants include the following:

Pacemakers: Sound baths that involve magnetic solid fields or intense vibrations could interfere with the functioning of pacemakers, which regulate the heart's electrical activity. Individuals with pacemakers need to consult with their healthcare provider to determine whether participating in sound baths is safe.

Cochlear implants: Vibrational therapy or intense sound vibrations may impact the functioning of cochlear implants, which are electronic devices that help individuals with hearing loss perceive sound. Those with cochlear implants must consult their healthcare provider before using sound baths to ensure no adverse effects.

Deep brain stimulation (DBS) devices: DBS devices are implanted to help manage certain neurological conditions, such as Parkinson's disease. Sound baths that involve magnetic fields or intense vibrations may interfere with the functioning of these devices. It is crucial to consult with a healthcare provider specializing in DBS to determine if sound baths are suitable or if any precautions need to be taken.

Implantable cardioverter-defibrillators (ICDs): ICDs are devices implanted in individuals at risk of life-threatening arrhythmias. Vibrational therapy or strong magnetic fields present in certain sound baths could interfere with the functioning of these devices.

Individuals with ICDs should consult their healthcare provider to determine whether sound baths are safe.

Neurostimulators: Neurostimulators, also known as spinal cord stimulators or nerve stimulators are implanted devices used for managing chronic pain or neurological conditions.

Sound baths that involve intense vibrations or magnetic fields may interfere with the functioning of these devices. Consultation with a healthcare provider specializing in neurostimulation is necessary to determine if sound baths are appropriate.

AFTERCARE

After experiencing a sound bath or vibrational therapy session, it is important to prioritize self-care and acknowledge that the healing process continues beyond the session, days beyond the session. The mind may feel more apparent, and the body may experience a release of tension and stress. Embrace this state of relaxation and allow yourself time to sit with it. Sound baths can enhance sensory perception, making you more attuned to your surroundings. You may notice subtle sounds, colors, or textures with greater clarity.

Sound therapy has the potential to stir emotions and release deeply held emotional patterns. After a session, you may experience various emotions, including joy, sadness, or even a sense of catharsis. Allow yourself to honor these emotions without judgment, providing yourself with a safe space for emotional processing.

Sound baths can help facilitate energy flow within the body, clearing energetic blockages. After a session, you might experience a renewed sense of power, inspiration, or motivation. You might also just feel tired and need to rest.

Allow yourself time for integration following the session. Engage in activities that promote relaxation, such as taking a bath, practicing gentle yoga or meditation, or spending time in nature. This will support the assimilation of the healing vibrations and promote a deeper integration of the experience.

Drink plenty of water after to aid in the release of toxins and maintain hydration.

Take time for self-reflection and journaling to explore any insights, emotions, or sensations that arose during the session. Writing down your experiences can deepen your understanding and provide a record of your healing.

Also prioritize healthy, whole foods that resonate with your body, such as fresh fruits and vegetables, Avoid heavy or processed foods that hinder the body's natural healing processes. Pairing sound baths with fasting, colon hydrotherapy, clean water, detoxes and rest can all help on your path of getting your body, mind and spirit back into its natural state which I will dive into deeper in further work.

Thank you all for reading and being a part of this journey :)

If you made it this far I appreciate you and the time you have taken to further your practice.

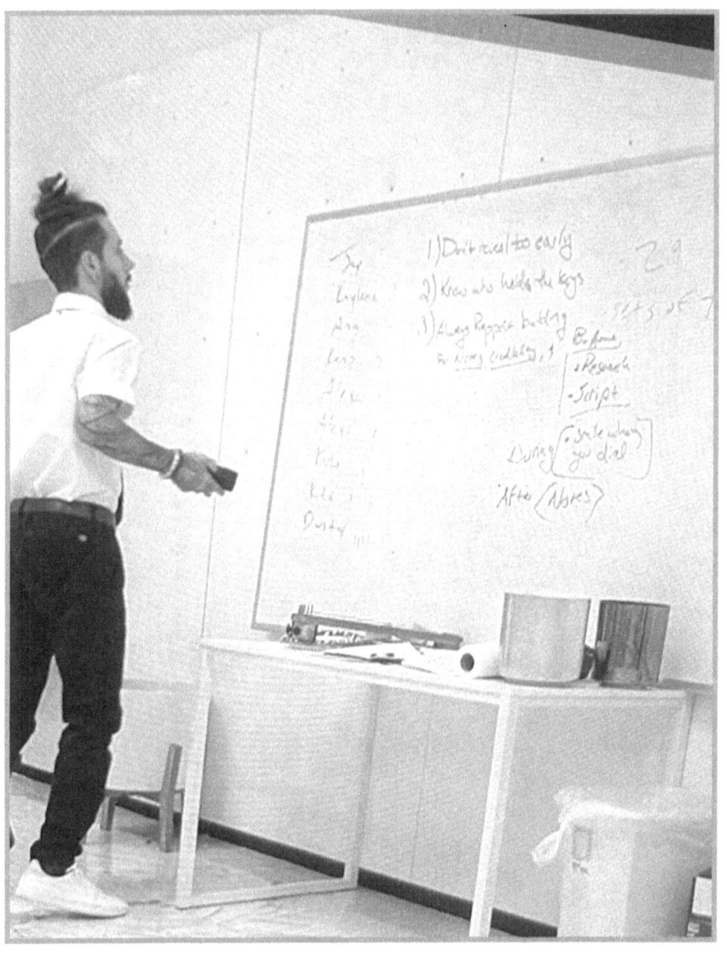

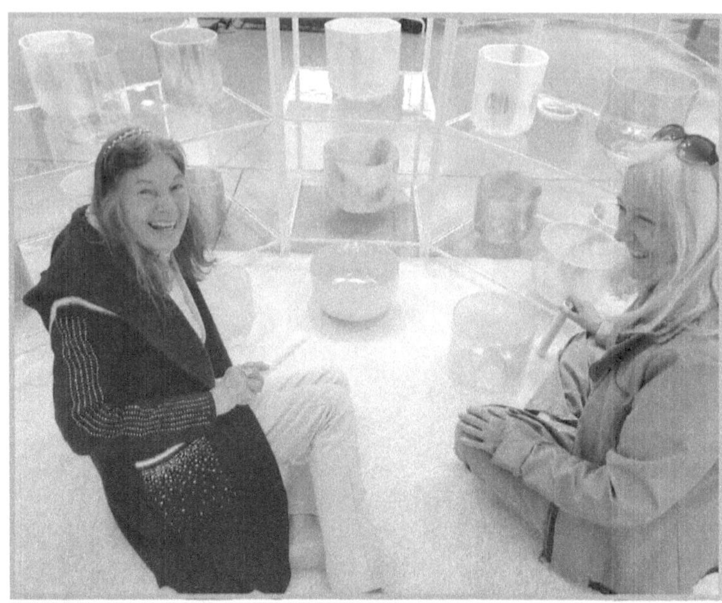

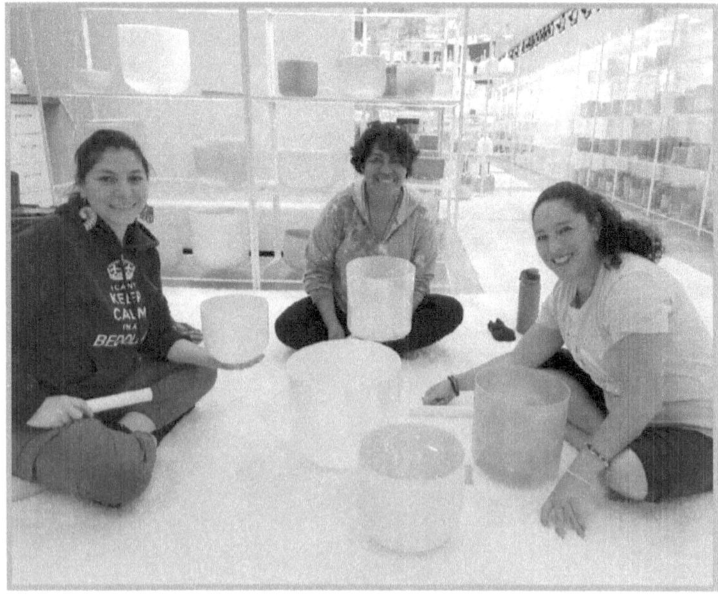

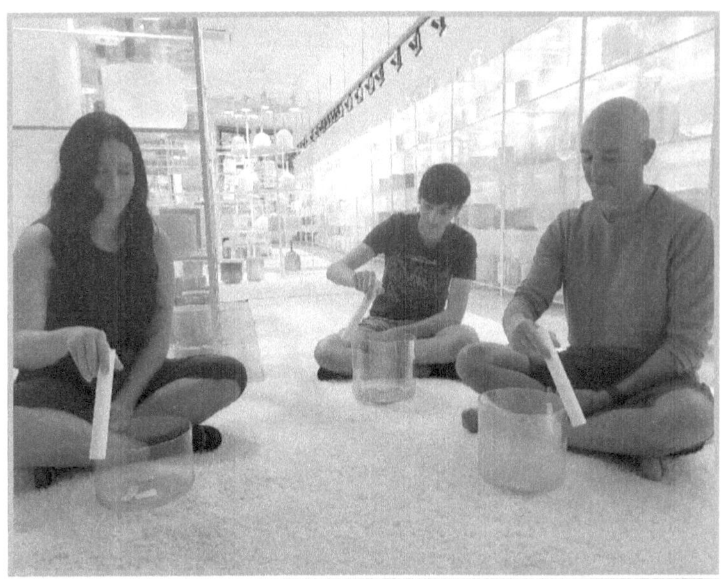

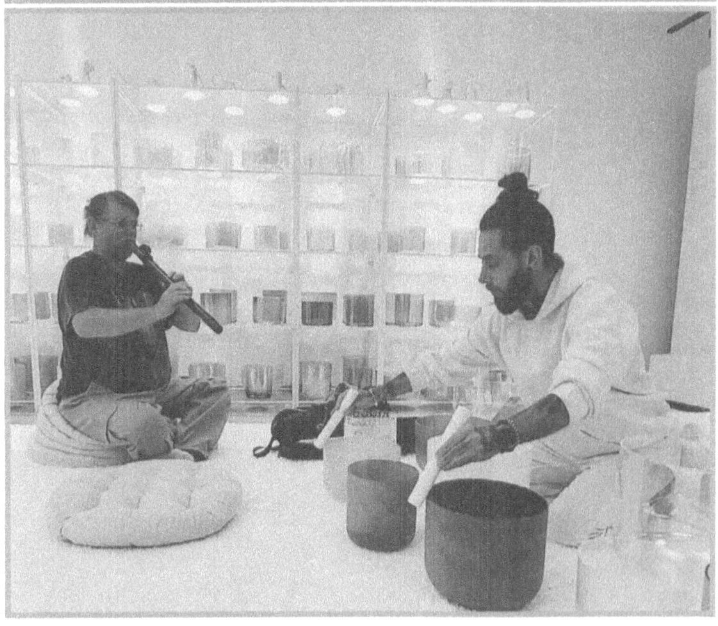

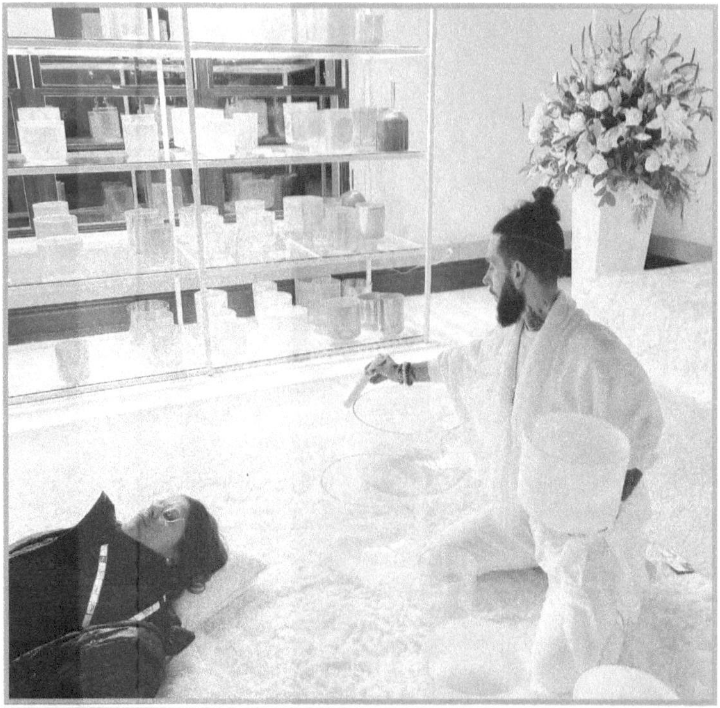

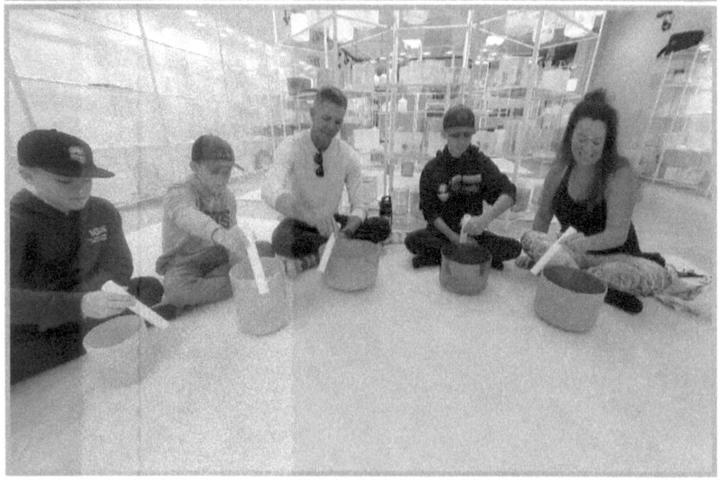

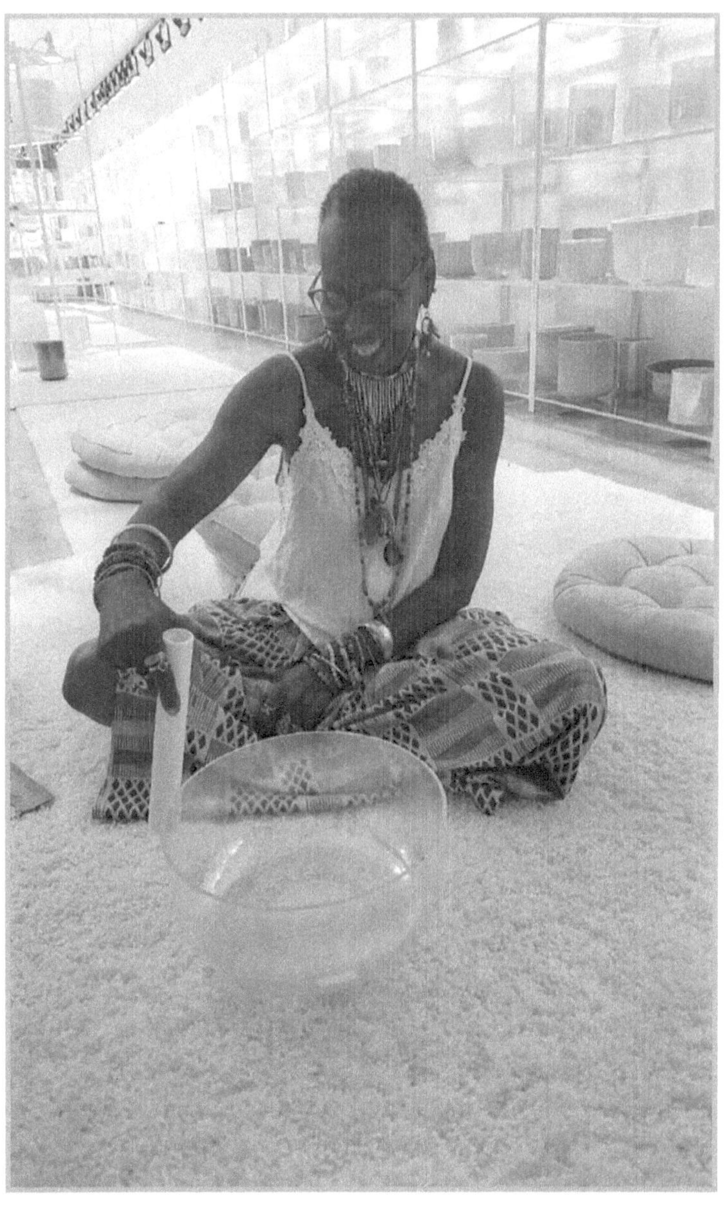

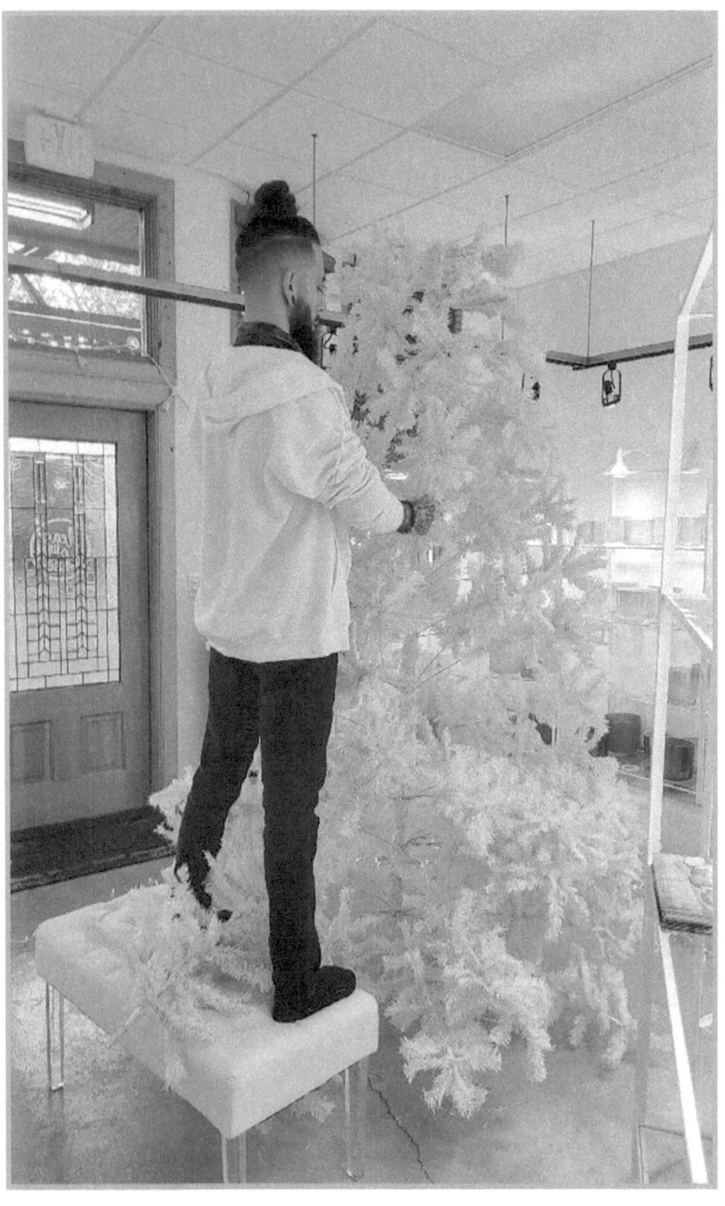

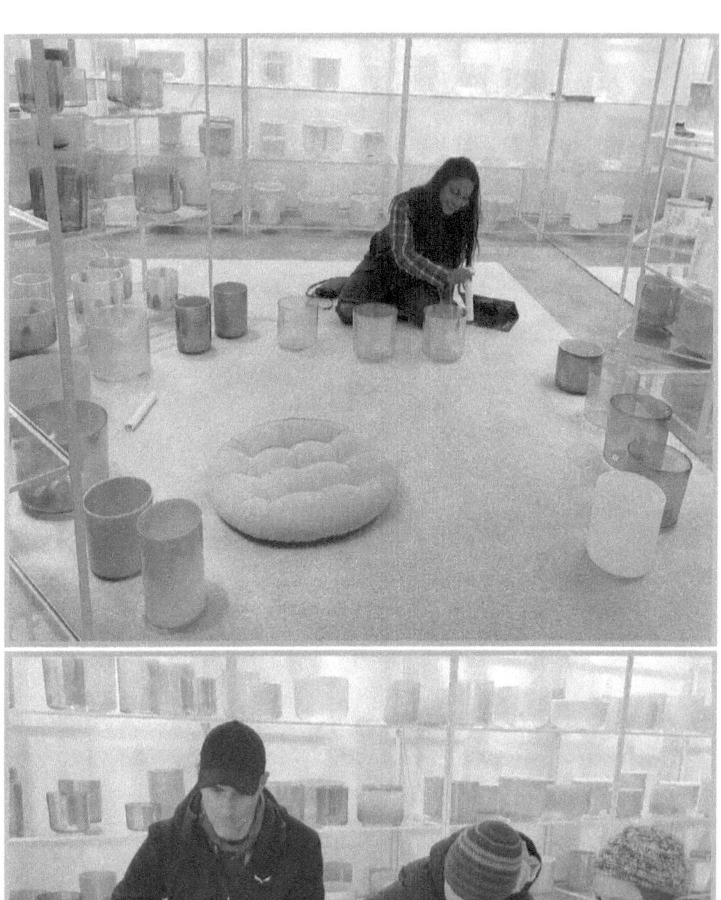

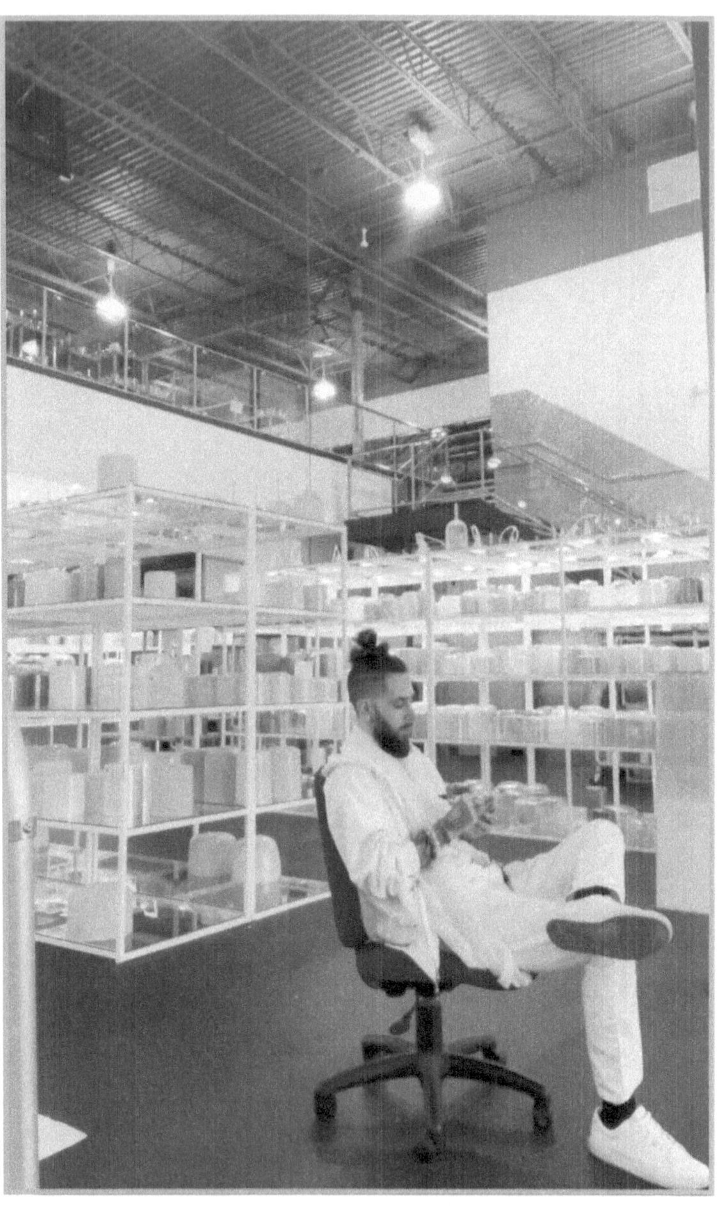

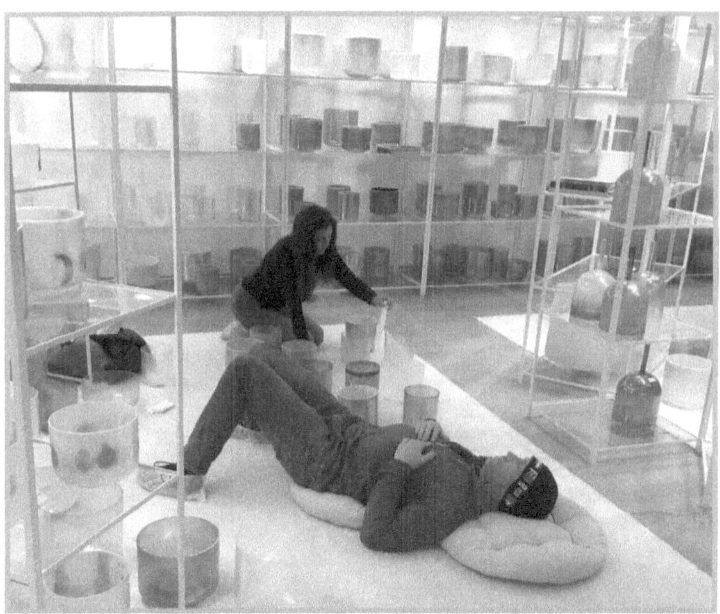

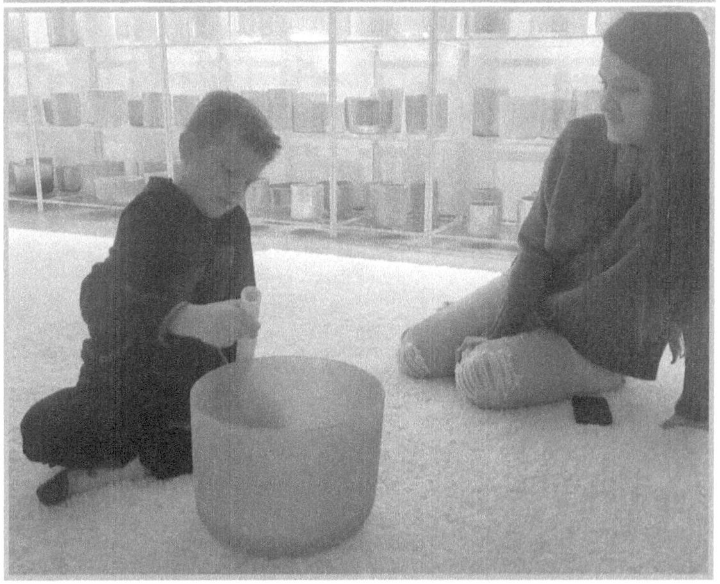

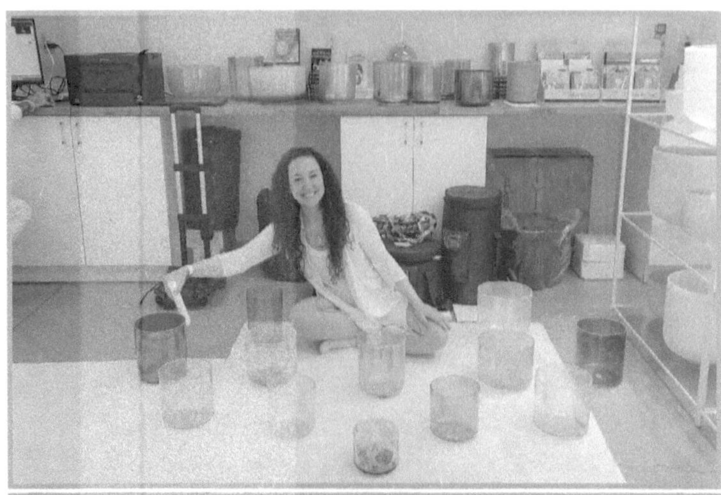

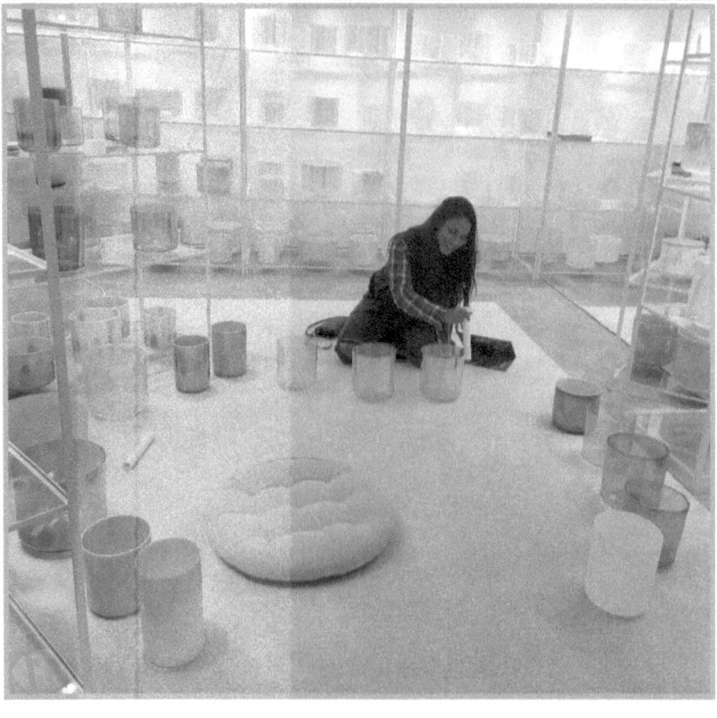

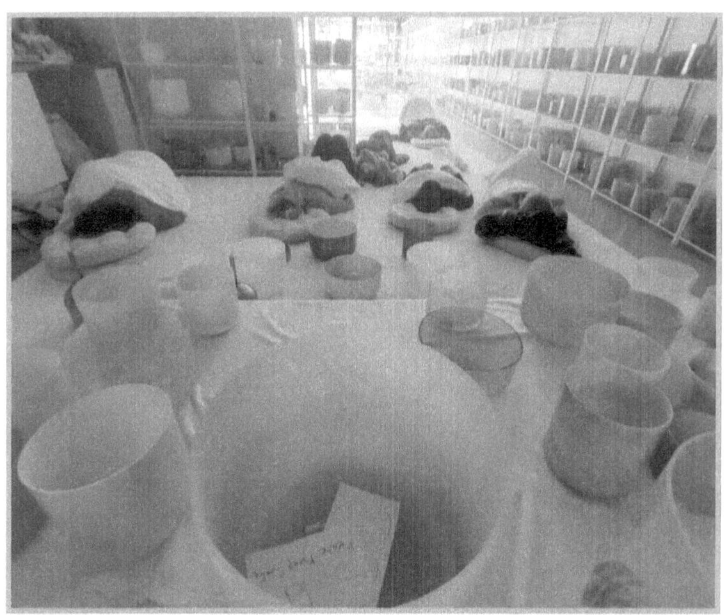

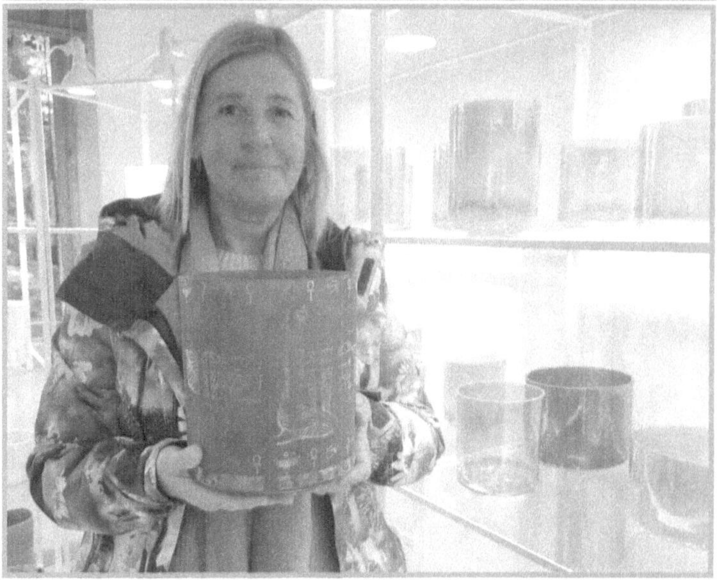

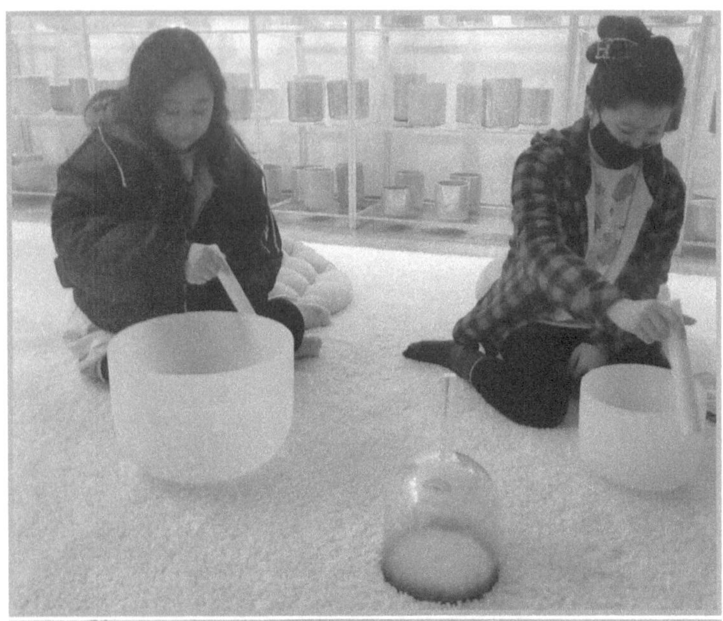

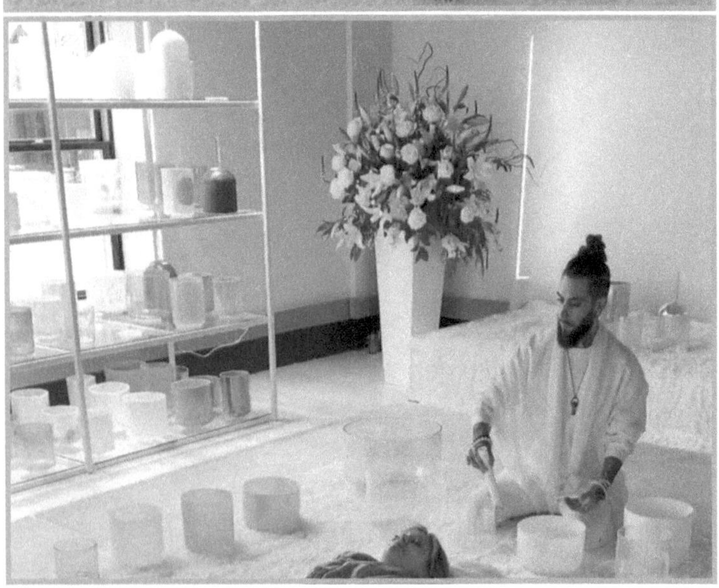

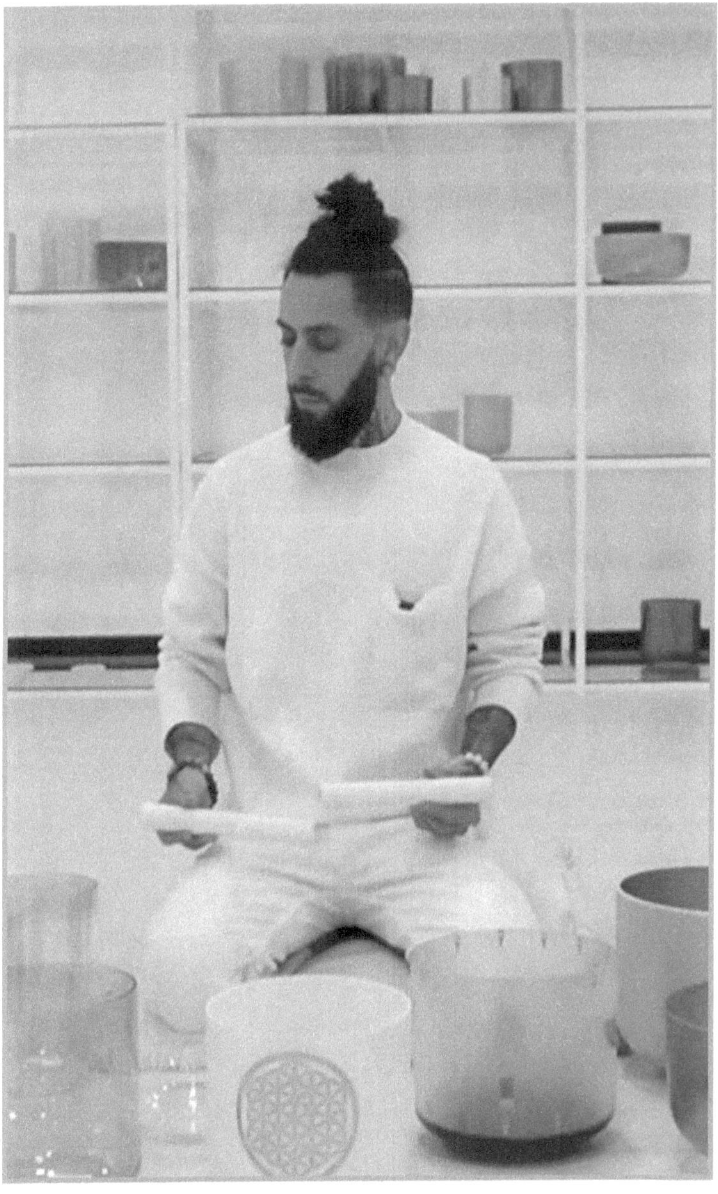

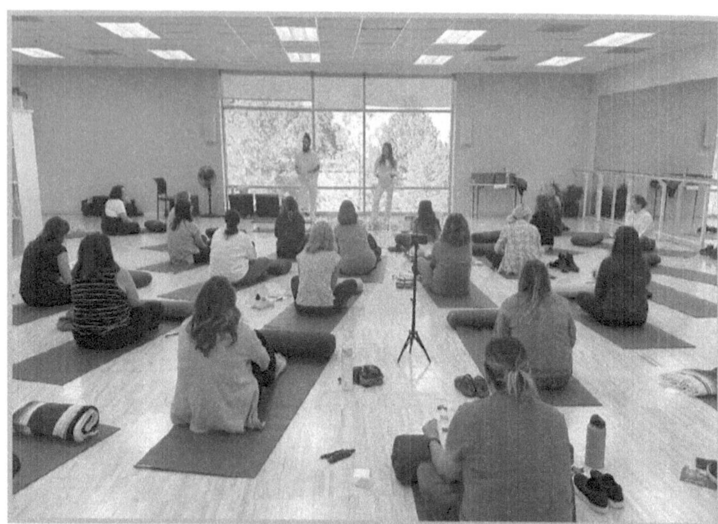

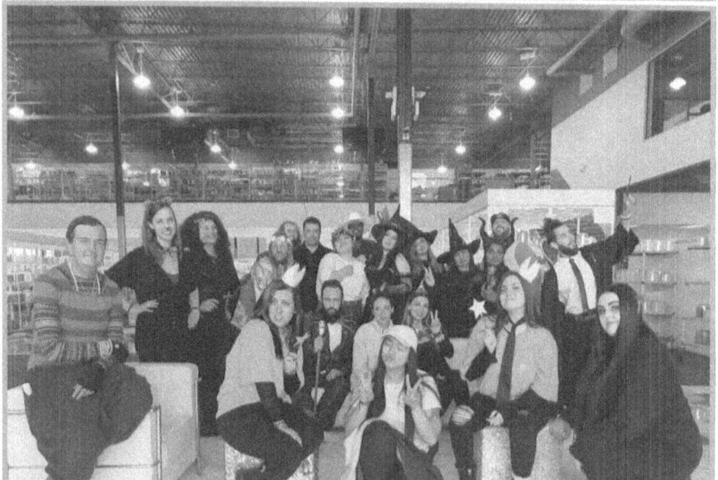

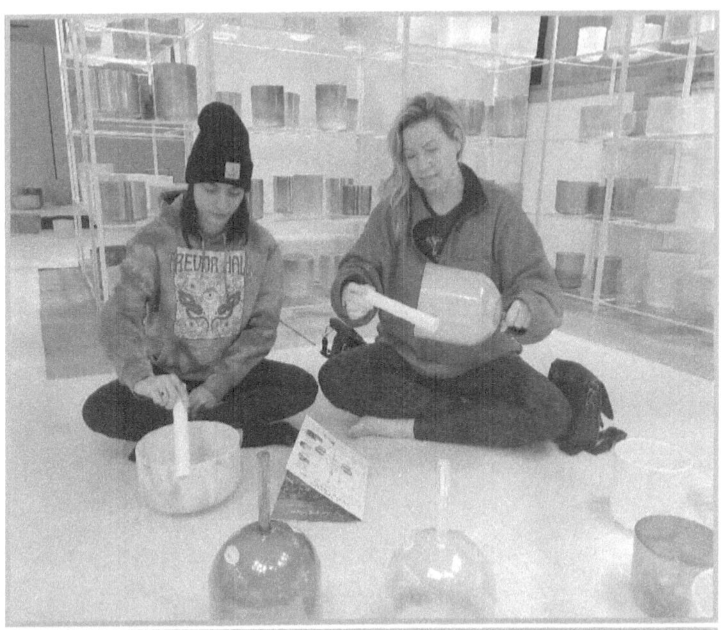

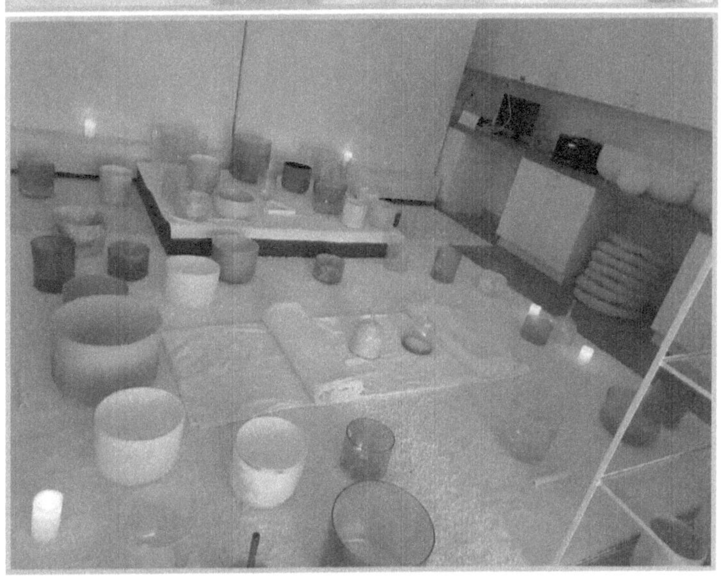

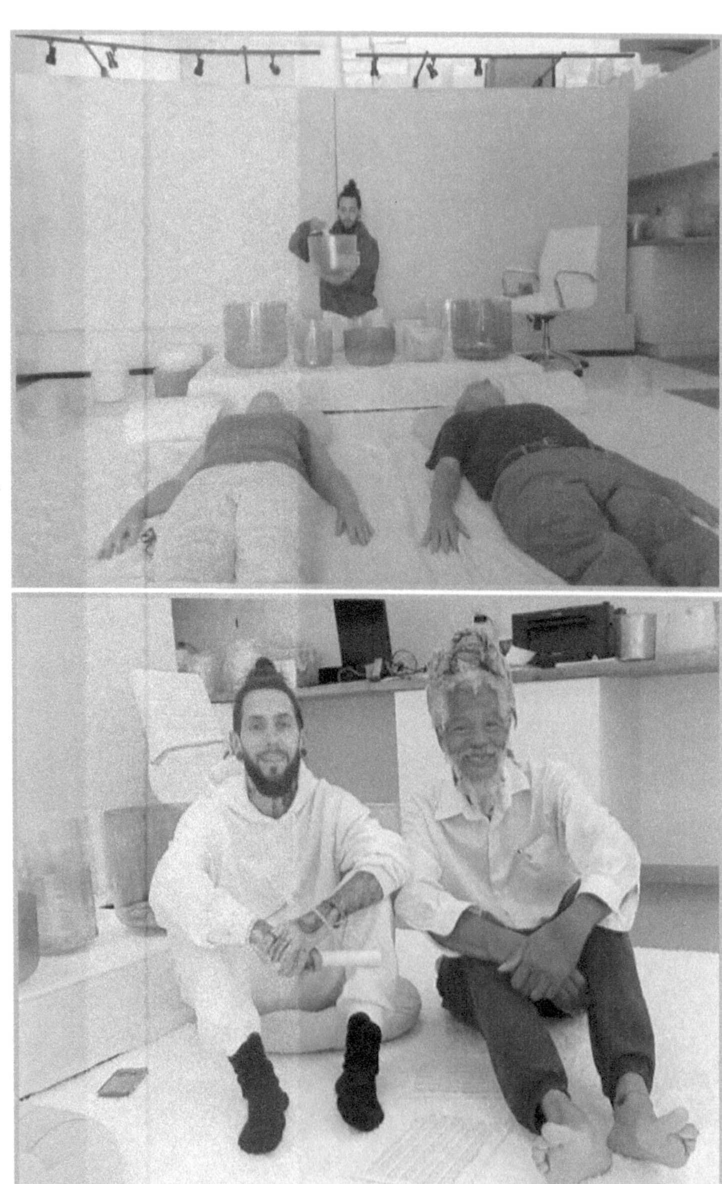

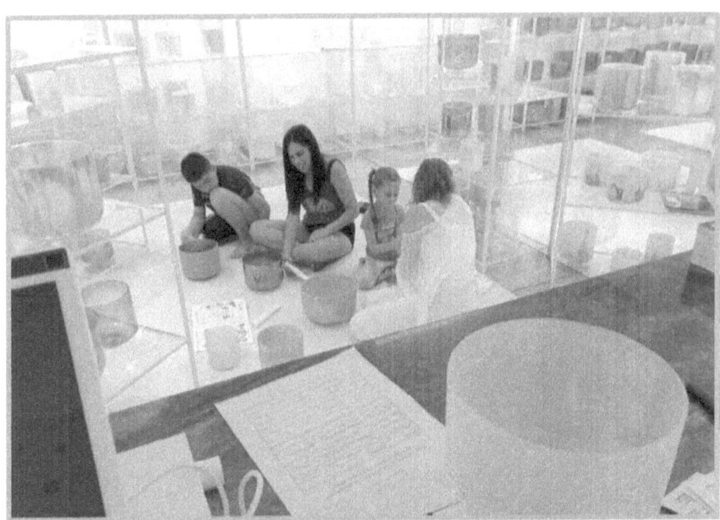

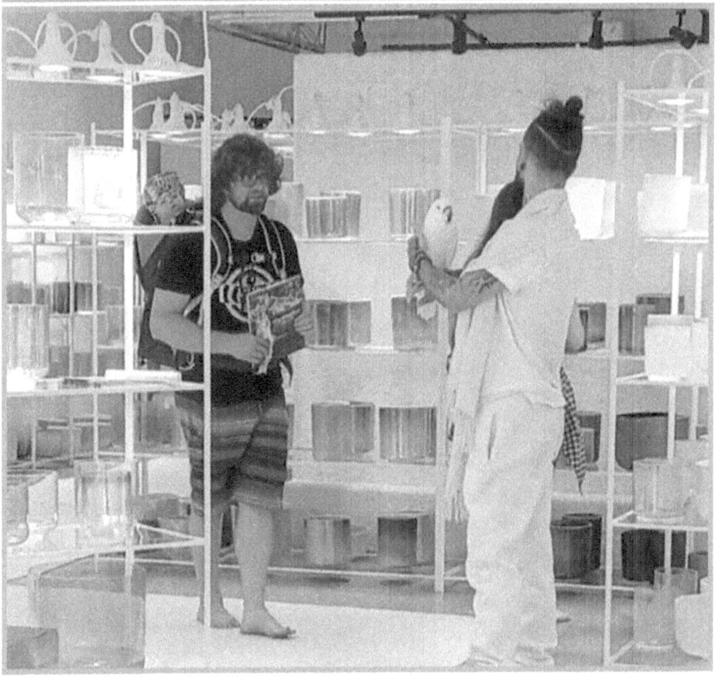

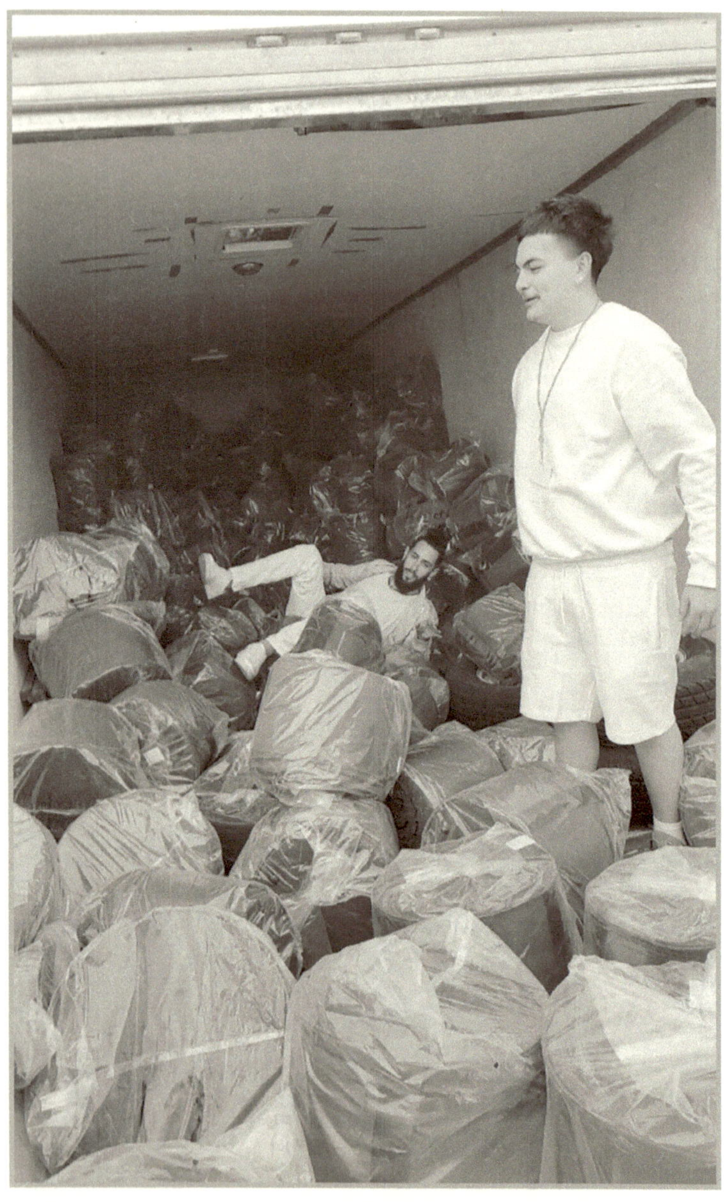

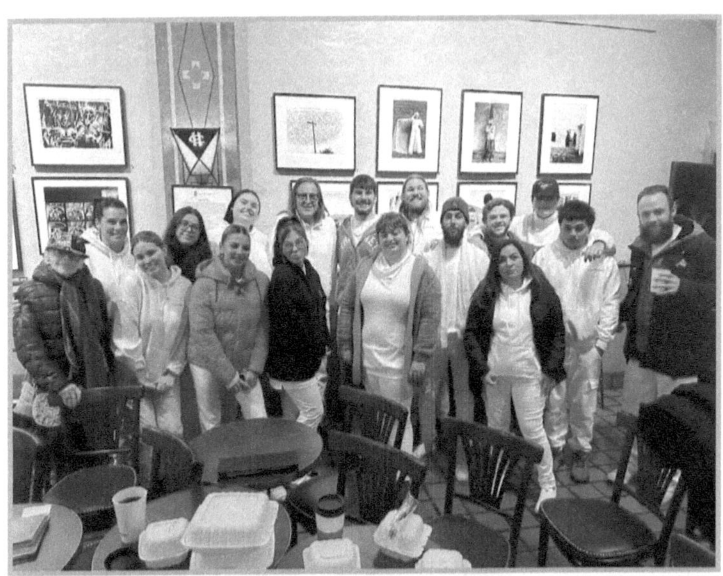

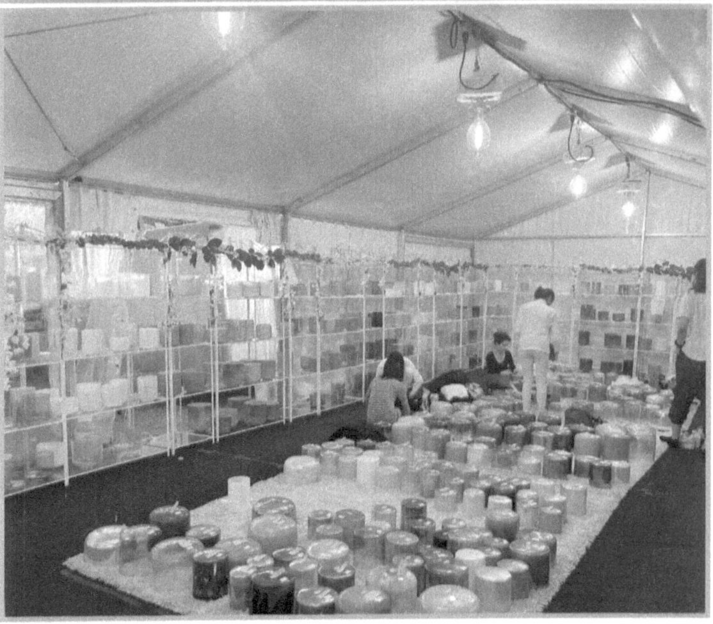

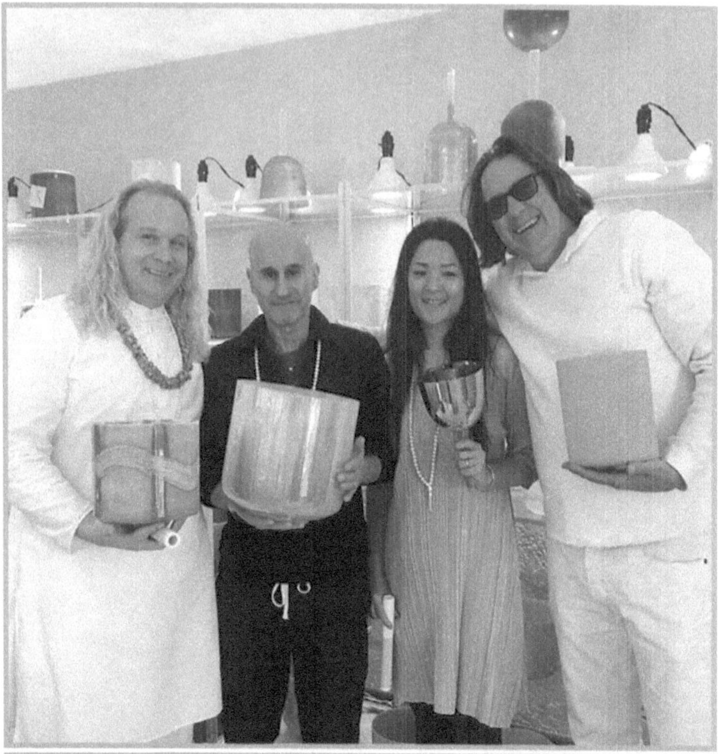

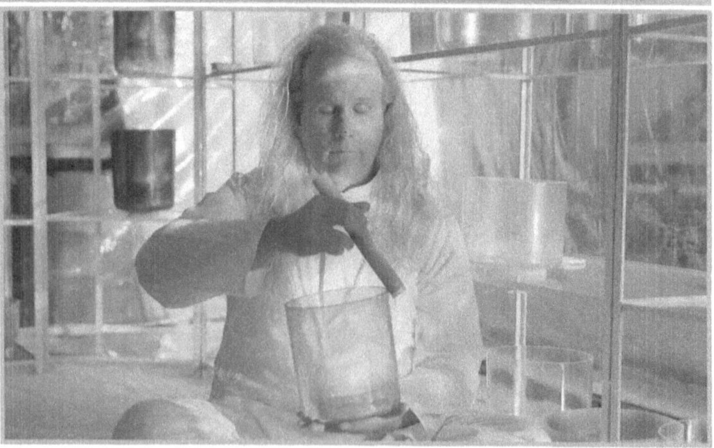

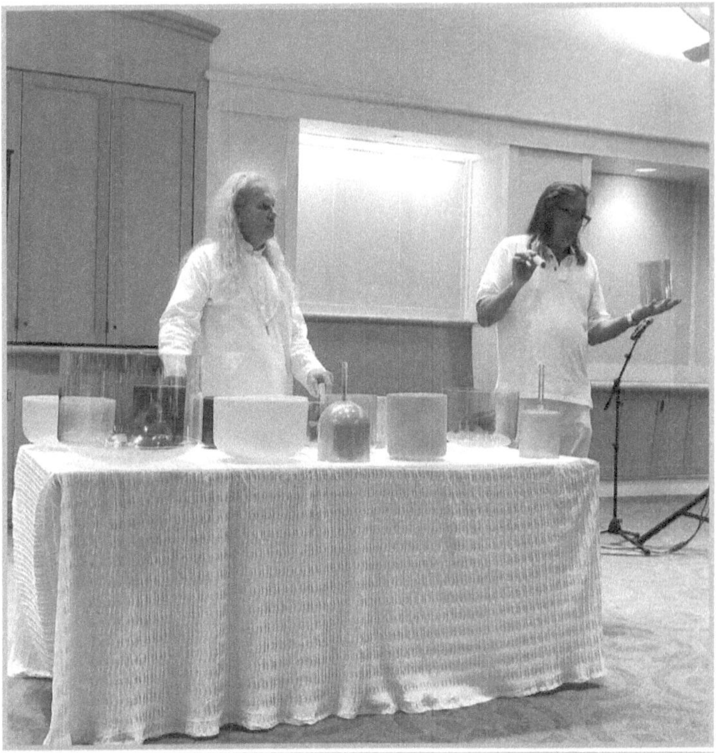

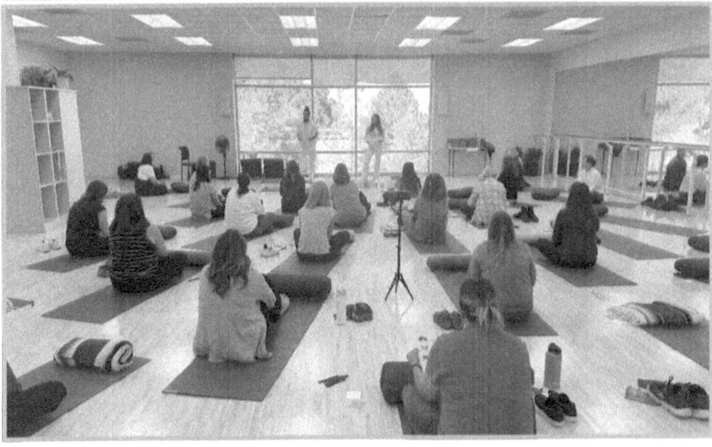

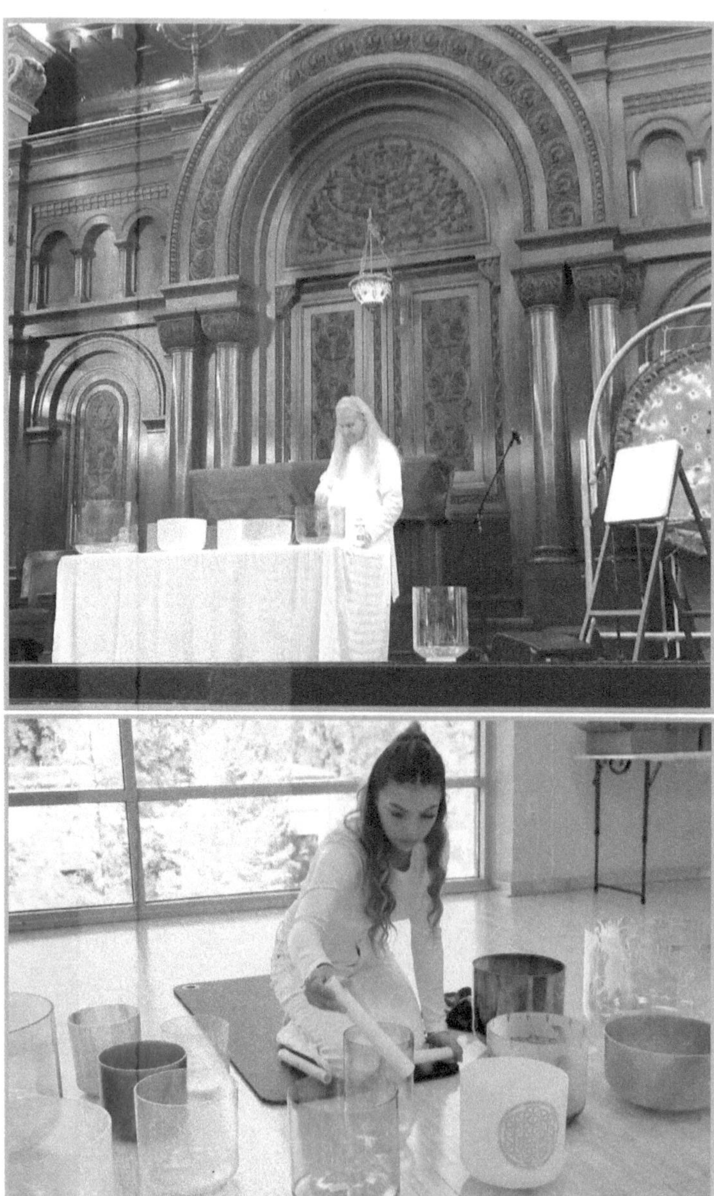

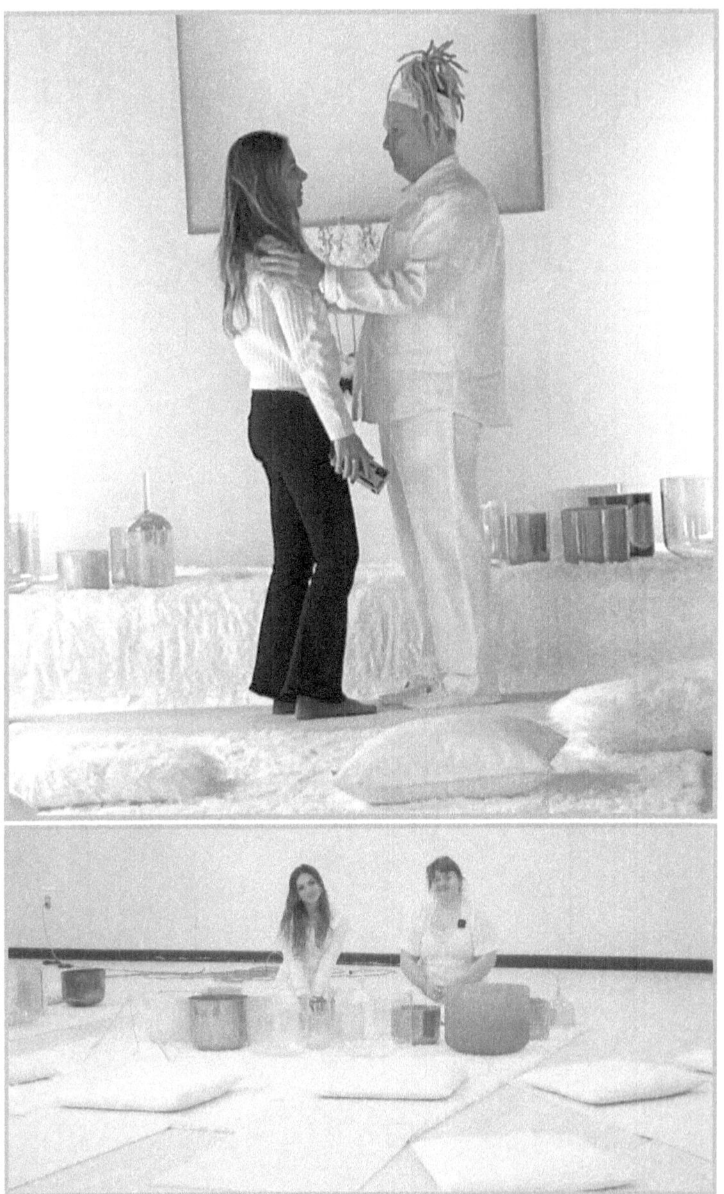

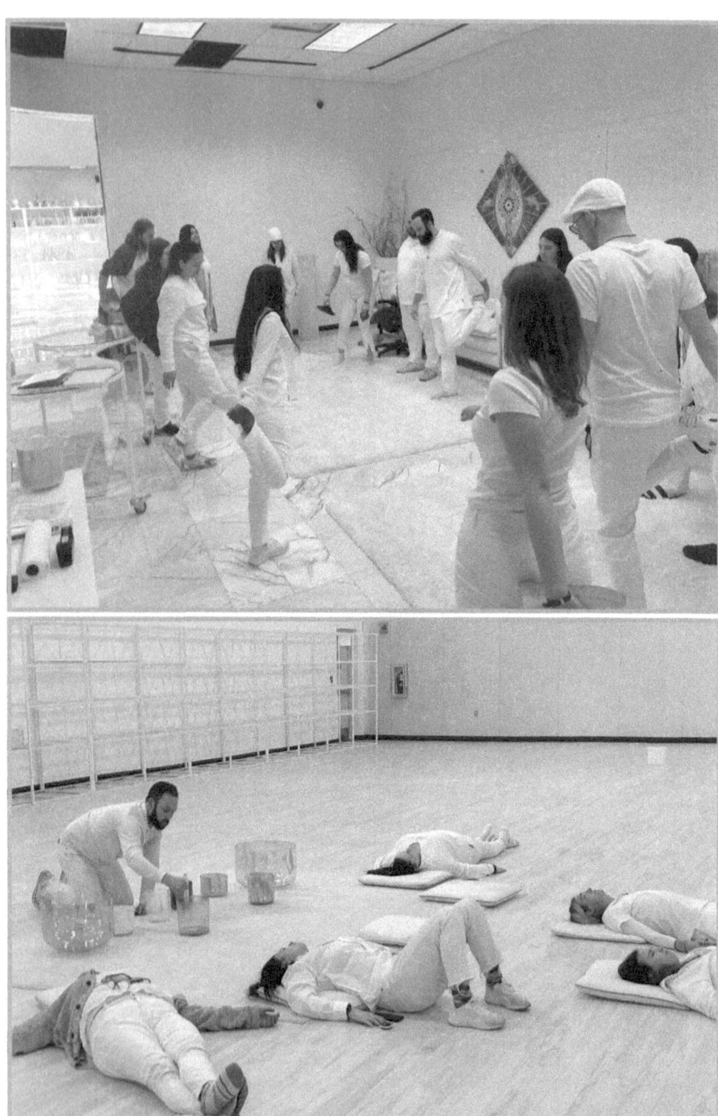

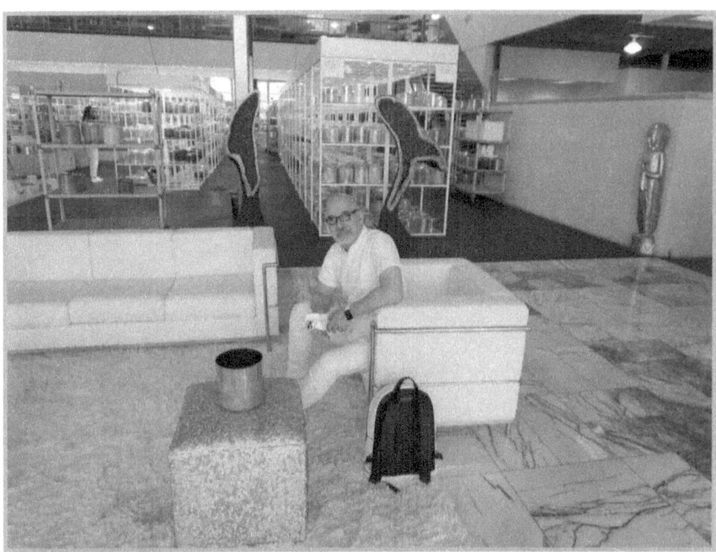

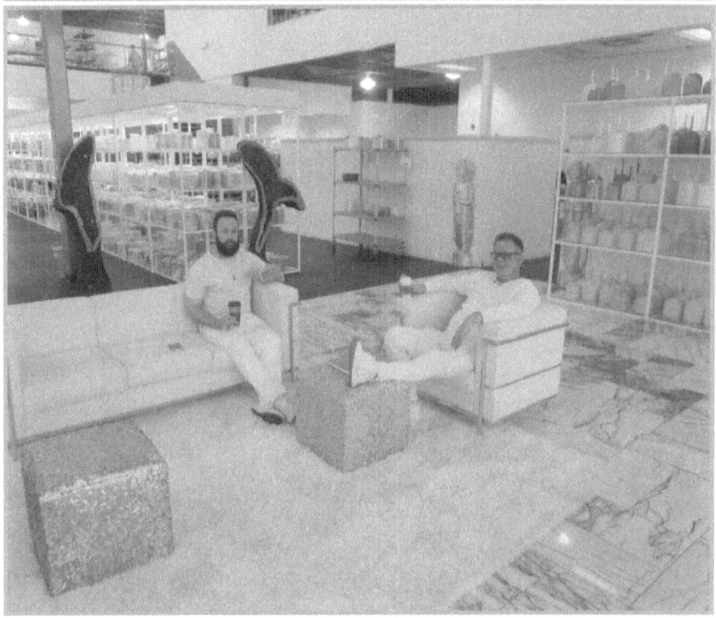

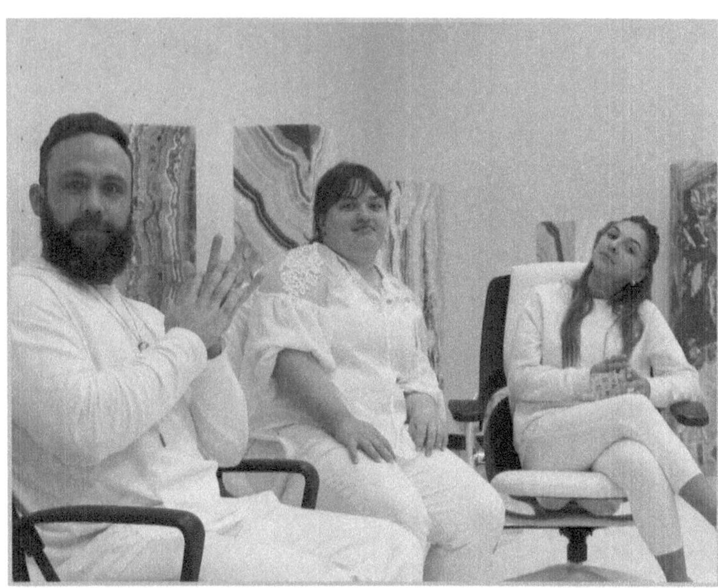

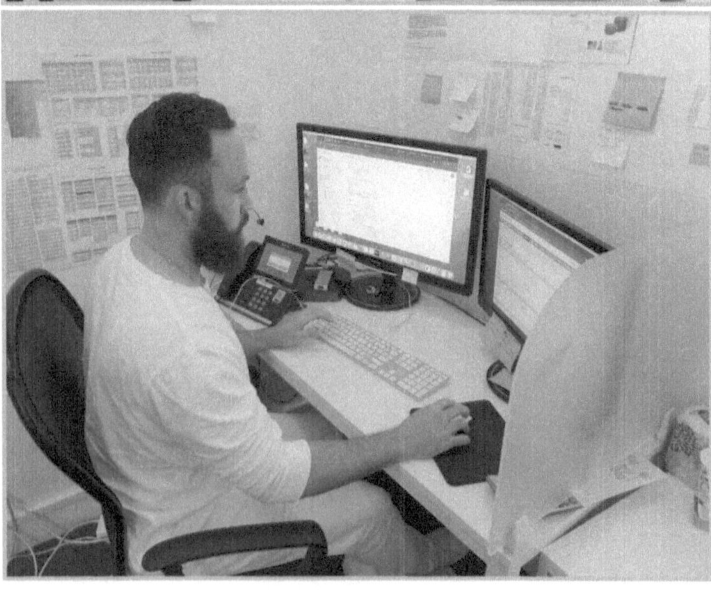

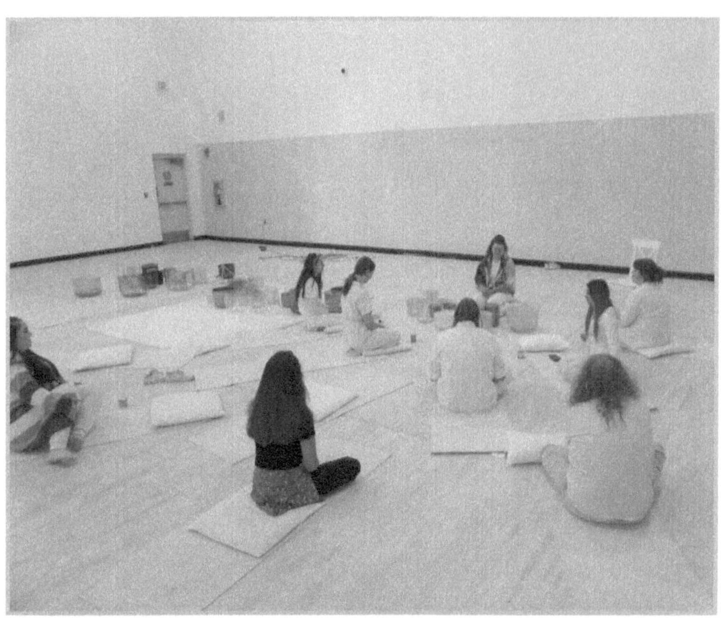

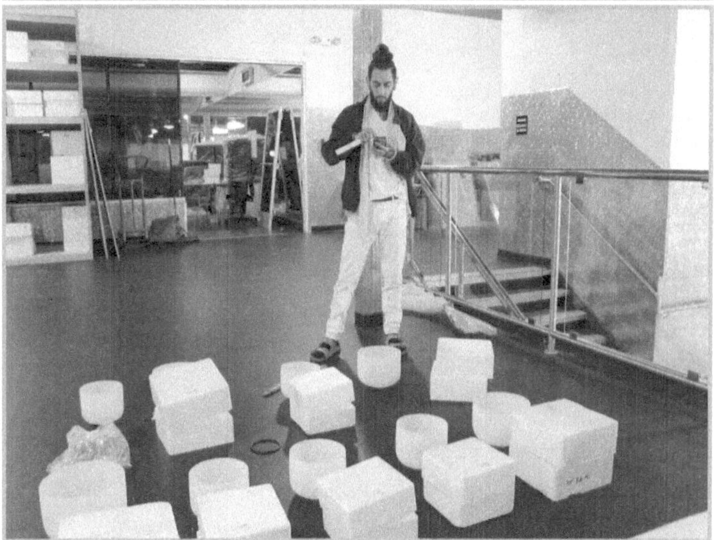

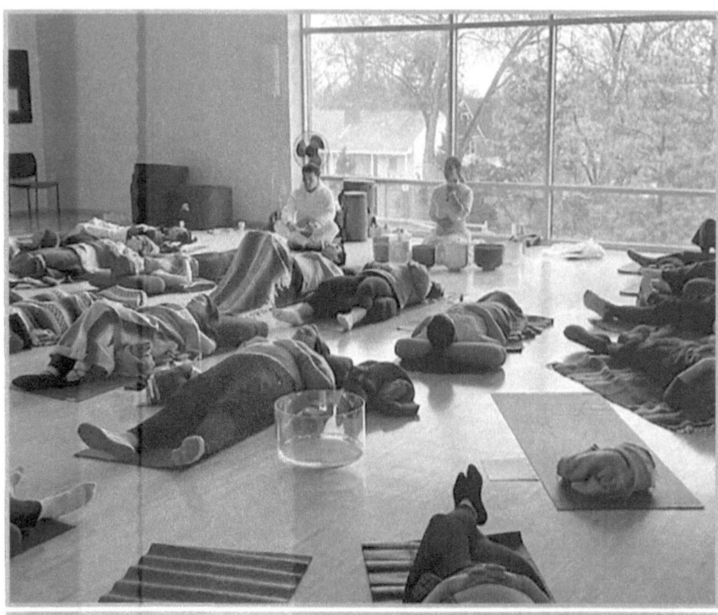

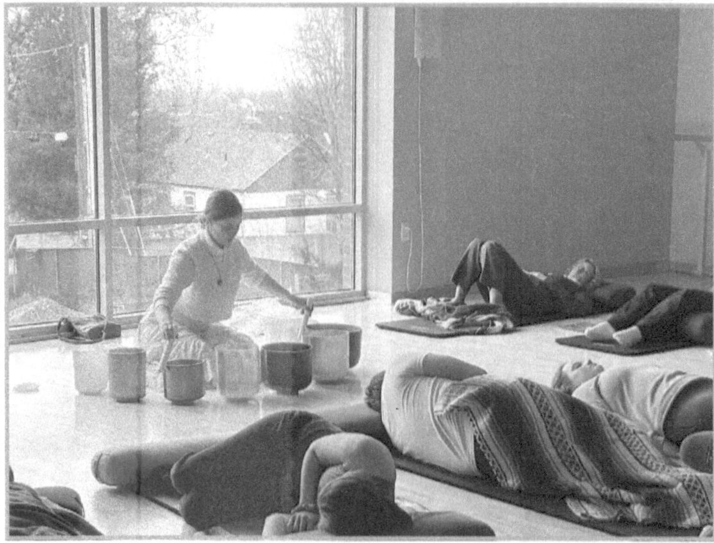

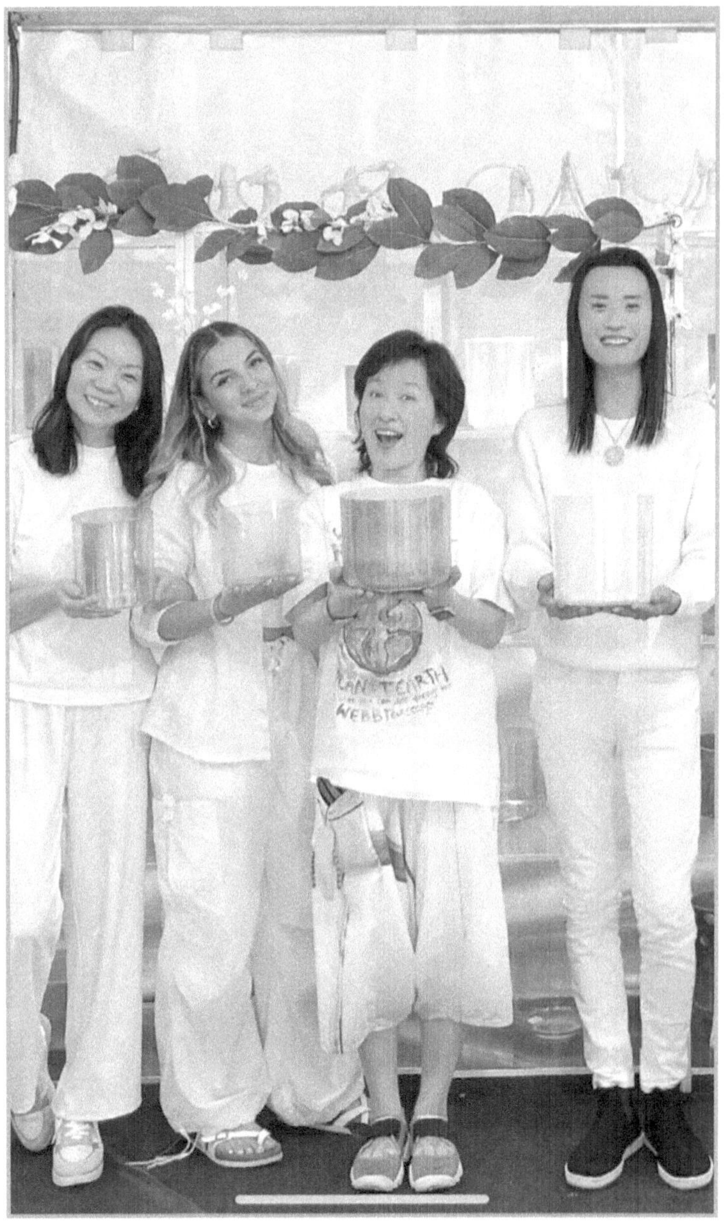

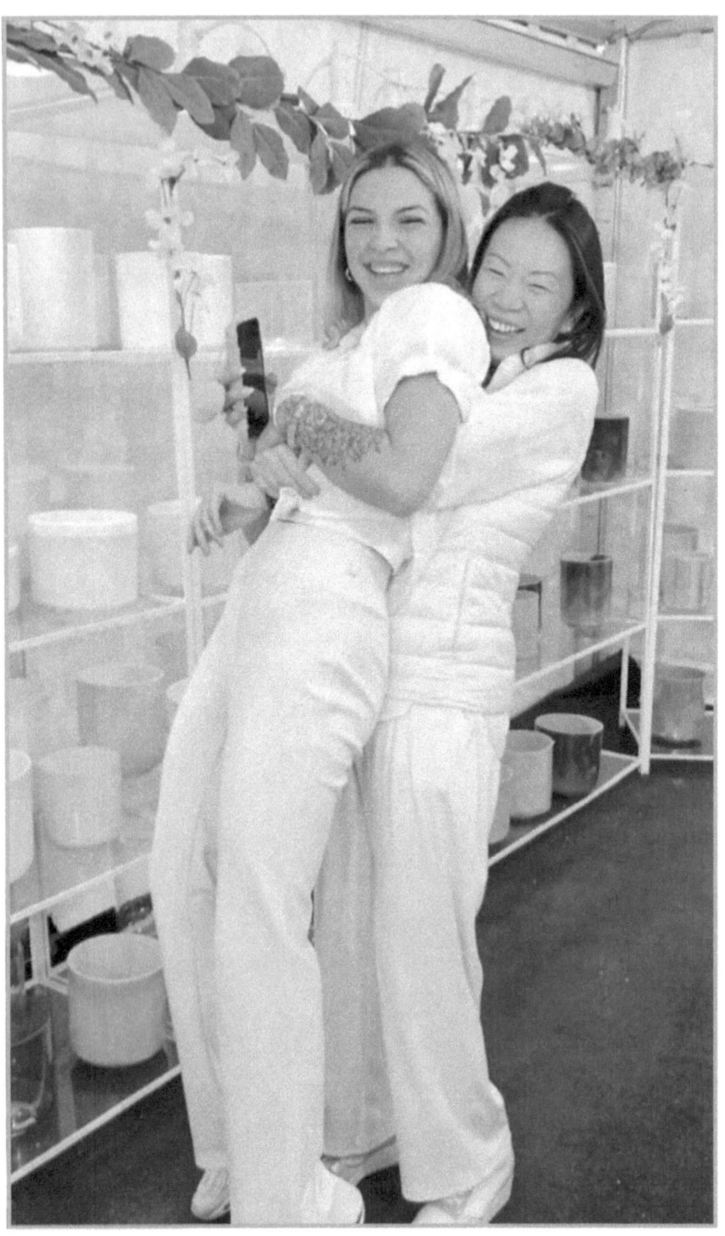

ABOUT THE AUTHOR

With an expanded yet humble understanding of sound healing, Jay Gibson has touched the lives of thousands, spending years working with Crystal Tones®, their extensive experience and testimonials speak volumes.

Jay's expertise is exceptional, as they have developed comprehensive curricula on sound healing and vibrational therapy with Crystal Bowls. Jay has helped thousands of Singing bowls find homes and continues to grow in his career. The standout achievement is Jay Gibson's creation of one of the most comprehensive resources for building sets with singing bowls. Jay's focus is to empower others through training, teachings, public speaking, sound baths and courses.

Jay Gibson, Founder of Know Thy Sound has experience working at rehab centers, providing assistance to troubled youth and volunteering at assisted living centers. In addition to spending the earlier part of his career in the music industry he excels at managing teams and empowering employees to unlock their full potential. Jay's sincere dedication to holistic health is evident in his work and personal practices.